Surgical Treatment of Ocular Inflammatory Disease

Joseph B. Michelson, M.D.
Head, Division of Ophthalmology
Director, Retina-Uveitis Service
Scripps Clinic and Research Foundation
La Jolla, California
Assistant Clinical Professor of Ophthalmology
University of California at San Diego School of Medicine
Consultant in Retina
United States Naval Regional Medical Center
San Diego, California

Robert A. Nozik, M.D.
Clinical Professor of Ophthalmology
University of California, San Francisco
Research Ophthalmologist
Francis I. Proctor Foundation for Research in Ophthalmology
San Francisco, California

With Contributions by

Mitchell H. Friedlaender, M.D.
Director, Cornea—External Disease Service
Division of Ophthalmology
Scripps Clinic and Research Foundation
La Jolla, California
Formerly Associate Clinical Professor of Ophthalmology
University of California
San Francisco, California

Ronald E. Smith, M.D.
Professor of Ophthalmology
University of Southern California
Estelle Doheny Eye Foundation
Los Angeles, California

Surgical Treatment of
Ocular Inflammatory Disease

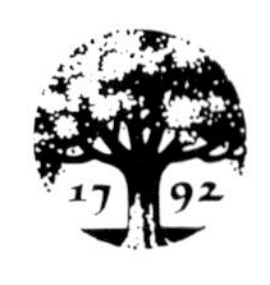

J. B. Lippincott Company *Philadelphia*
London Mexico City New York
St. Louis São Paulo Sydney

Acquisitions Editor: Lisette Bralow
Sponsoring Editor: Sanford Robinson
Design Coordinator: Michelle Gerdes
Production Manager: Carol A. Florence
Production Coordinator: Kathryn Rule
Compositor: TAPSCO, Inc.
Printer/Binder: Murray Printing Company

1 3 5 6 4 2

Library of Congress Cataloging-in-Publication Data

Michelson, Joseph B.
Surgical treatment of ocular inflammatory disease.

Includes bibliographies and index.
1. Uveitis—Surgery. 2. Eye—Inflammation.
3. Eye—Surgery. I. Nozik, Robert A. (Robert Alan),
DATE. II. Title. [DNLM: 1. Eye—surgery.
2. Uveitis—complications. 3. Uveitis—surgery.
WW 240 M623s]
RE351.M55 1988 617.7'2059 87-34246
ISBN 0-397-50763-1

The authors and publisher have exerted every effort to ensure that drug selection and dosage set forth in this text are in accord with current recommendations and practice at the time of publication. However, in view of ongoing research, changes in government regulations, and the constant flow of information relating to drug therapy and drug reactions, the reader is urged to check the package insert for each drug for any change in indications and dosage and for added warnings and precautions. This is particularly important when the recommended agent is a new or infrequently employed drug.

This book is dedicated to G. Richard O'Connor, whose inspiring scholarship and dedicated teaching have influenced an entire generation of ophthalmologists.

Preface

Surgical Treatment of Ocular Inflammatory Disease began as an outgrowth of our chapter, "Uveitis Surgery," which appeared in Duane's five-volume text *Clinical Ophthalmology*. At the outset, we realized that it was impossible to condense all of the recent medical and surgical information, innovation, and instrumentation pertinent to uveitis diagnosis and treatment into one chapter. At the publisher's request, we considered an expanded volume to do just that. The result is now before you. Although inflammatory disease is an important part of so many current ophthalmology textbooks, there is no other text in which the surgical considerations and options are central to the perspective of uveitis alone.

Uveitis has always been a diagnostic mystery and therapeutic challenge. Ophthalmologists had previously desired to simplify it in order to lessen its confusion. We now live in a time that permits us the technological luxury to do the opposite. By studying its complexity, separating out its many specific disease syndromes and peculiar manifestations, we can offer patients treatment and options, and hence, cures, that heretofore did not exist. The strategies for cataract removal, for example, differ in juvenile rheumatoid arthritis, Fuch's heterochromic cyclitis, and "burned out" pars planitis. The whole spectrum of intra-ocular lens implantation and inflammatory conditions is ever-changing, as is the spectrum of inflammation in normal eyes caused by intra-ocular lenses themselves. The strategy for retinal detachment repair, for example, is different for traction detachment in pars planitis than it is for a combined traction and rheg-

ONE

Introduction

Until recently little has been written about the surgical management of the patient with uveitis because of the many failures with complicated surgical uveitis. The lack of success has been complicated by the belief that uveitis is a single disease cluster and that its diagnosis could be determined only with the greatest difficulty. Moreover, there were no special surgical procedures or even major modifications of standard techniques to counteract glaucoma, retinal detachment, or vitreal opacifications in the patient with uveitis.

Recently, remarkable progress has been made. Using a systematic approach, the general ophthalmologist should be able to diagnose properly at least 80% of patients with uveitis. Unquestionably, accurate diagnosis is essential in determining what is the most appropriate treatment. All of the options allowed by the natural history and progression of the disease entity must be taken into account before surgical intervention is considered. It should be kept in mind that not all uveitic entities will respond identically to a specific form of intervention; the chance for success of a procedure therefore is directly related to the correct assignment of a patient to a specific diagnostic category.

Let us examine some of the considerations that have direct bearing on the decision of whether to operate, what procedure to use, and what medical measures to take preoperatively, during surgery, and postoperatively.

Surgery should not be undertaken until the eye has been free of uveitic activity for a prolonged period. The best time to operate is after the active inflammatory phase of the uveitis has burned out. This may be particularly true in cases of pars planitis or intermediate uveitis, for example, where the natural history of the disease suggests an endpoint to the inflammatory phase. If this is not practical, the next best time to operate is when the uveitis has been inactive for several months without treatment with corticosteroids. This is true in those cases of acute intermittent inflammation such as ankylosing spondylitis or Reiter's disease. If even this is not possible, then corticosteroids with an immunosuppressant should be used to quiet the eye as much as possible for at least a month before surgery. In some situations, the ongoing inflammation is chronic and unrelenting, and the surgical procedure may be necessary to relieve or reduce part of the uveitic problem, as in endophthalmitis or toxoplasmic retinal detachment.

In order to reduce the manipulation of diseased or inflamed tissue, the approach should be through a normal entry wherever possible. For example, if the primary inflammatory site is in the anterior uvea, surgery through a posterior approach may be preferable. Conversely, if the primary inflammatory site is posterior, then the anterior approach is optimum.

Uveitic entities in which there is little or no tendency to develop anterior or posterior synechiae (e.g., pars planitis, Fuchs' heterochromic iridocyclitis) respond to surgical intervention much better than "sticky" uveitic entities (e.g., sarcoid, chronic iridocyclitis of juvenile rheumatoid arthritis). Acute recurrent uveitic eyes tolerate surgery better than chronically uveitic eyes.

Uveitis in association with a markedly low intra-ocular pressure (prephthisical), especially in the absence of a cyclitic membrane, may indicate that the eye is a poor surgical risk. The removal of a cyclitic membrane, however, may restore a prephthisical eye to a higher pressure and confer a more positive prognosis.

The pre-operative, operative, and postoperative use of local, systemic, or periocular corticosteroids allows the uveitic eye to tolerate intra-ocular surgery better.

This text presents an overview of the surgical treatment of ocular inflammatory disease, including the general measures and specific indications for surgical intervention in this complicated situation. One must consider the time and approach for surgical intervention and, more specifically, those disease states which require precise knowledge of their inflammatory behavior. Later chapters discuss pre-operative, intra-operative, and postoperative medications for all of the ocular inflammatory diseases, including those which fall in the spectrum of herpetic bacterial and fungal keratouveitis and retinitis as well as endophthalmitis. Difficult diagnostic and surgical considerations for septic emboli to the eye are discussed, as are the ever-increasing and frequent problem of drug-abuse type endophthalmitis. A detailed chapter on the immunology of ocular inflammation is also included.

The chapter on paracentesis of the eye includes a detailed listing of the antigen, antibody, direct and indirect immunofluorescent antibody techniques, such as enzyme immunoassay, enzyme-linked immunosorbent assay, complement fractions, immunodiffusion, and indirect hemoglutination tests. For many infectious organisms found in the aqueous and vitreous, this is probably the most up-to-date compilation of serology testing for intra-ocular inflammations measured in microtiter quantities. In addition, the discussion of diagnostic paracentesis outlines the findings of tumor cells, eosinophils, microphages, bacteria, and fungi seen in intra-ocular inflammatory disease. Specific instructions on how to retrieve samples and prepare slides is included. This chapter presents material at the cutting edge of intra-ocular diagnosis for both medical and surgical ocular inflammatory disease.

A complete discussion of the corneal manifestations of ocular inflammatory disease, with its necessary surgery for active corneal decompensation, is included. This encompasses a discussion of the herpetic infections of the eye: when, where, and how, more specifically, to proceed with corneal transplantation. When these very common and yet devastating infectious diseases affect the eye, uveitic glaucoma presents a unique challenge for the clinician. The underlying etiology for all of the glaucomas with uveitic conditions is inflammatory. The handling of posterior synechiae may be very different from the simple medical management of posterior synechiae with a pupillary block. The treatment of iris bombé may be very different from that of peripheral synechiae, which may or may not complicate an inflammatory "trabeculitis."

The range of uveitic glaucoma is discussed with pointed references to the clinical features and pathology of inflammatory intra-ocular pressure elevations. Specific note is taken of Posner-Schlossman syndrome, herpes simplex and herpes zoster uveitis, severe or acute iridocyclitis, Fuchs' heterochromic cyclitis, mechanisms of blockage of the trabeculum with debris, peripheral anterior synechiae, trabeculitis, rubeosis iridis, hypersecretion syndromes, and sclerosis of the cortical meshwork. Special mention is made of traumatic glaucoma, as well, which ushers in a whole different set of considerations along with hemorrhagic glaucoma, foreign body inflammation, and infection in the eye with siderosis. This is treated in the glaucoma section as well as in the retinal detachment and trauma sections. While lens-induced glaucoma and lens-induced uveitis are uncommon, their clinical picture can be so specific and their clinical outcome so devastating that they deserve special mention.

A very important topic to be considered in the treatment of ocular inflammatory disease is cataract extraction in specific uveitic syndromes. Cataract extractions pose significant risks for patients with uveitis. The outcome of cataract surgery depends heavily upon the particular uveitic syndrome. In many uveitis syndromes, a cataract may be caused by the inflammation itself, which produces significant lens opacity, or by the chronic use of corticosteroids which, of course, may cause cataracts. It is generally agreed that an eye that has been quiet without medications and has been free of active inflammation for a long time usually poses the least risk for cataract surgery. However, there are situations in which cataract surgery is necessary and the inflammation in the eye is present or minimal but must be dealt with accordingly.

The earliest results of extracapsular cataract extraction in patients with juvenile rheumatoid arthritis were discouraging, owing to the frequent loss of vitreous, incarcerations into the wound, and the consequent development of cyclitic membrane with the subsequent development of ciliary body detachment and eventual phthisis. With the advent of the lensectomy-vitrectomy surgery using modern vitrectomy instruments, this is no longer the case and the cyclitic membrane can be entirely extirpated, leaving the ciliary body without detachment or traction, thus greatly lessening the potential for eventual hypotension and phthisis in these eyes. Other specific uveitic syndromes, such as pars planitis or intermediate uveitis and Fuchs' heterochromic iridocyclitis, do well with cataract extraction (cataract development is an integral part of the late stages of Fuchs' heterochromic iridocyclitis along with glaucoma). There are a few specific situations in which intra-ocular lens placement is not contraindicated in uveitis, Fuchs' heterochromic iridocyclitis being one of the generally accepted ones. In general, the implantation of intra-ocular lenses is contraindicated in active uveitis and should only be considered in cases that are "burned out," as when pars planitis eventually becomes quiescent of its own natural history.

Uveitis may be a consequence of cataract surgery itself, since inflammation in the early postoperative period following either cataract surgery or intra-ocular lens implantation may, in part, be related to surgical manipulation. What occurs is a response to change in breakdown of the blood aqueous barrier or to retained lens material, following extracapsular cataract extraction, or to tissue damage itself. Some surgeons have even postulated an "immunologic" inflammation due to the implant material. Some of this persistent type of intra-ocular inflammation may be minimized or reduced by prostaglandin inhibitors such as indomethacin, nonsteroidal agents, or aspirin. The retained lens material usually causes an inflammatory response that is transient and mild, and only in rare cases will it be prolonged, significant, or necessitate surgical removal. The incidence of this type of transient iridocyclitis following extracapsular surgery has decreased markedly from the early days of intra-ocular lens implantation. Interestingly, most studies have shown that infectious endophthalmitis does not occur with a higher frequency after intraocular lens implantation than one might anticipate following simple cataract removal.

We have witnessed, with the advent of the most modern extracapsular extractions with intra-ocular lens implantations, a lessening of many of the fears of postoperative infection that were present earlier with the more bulky and clumsy surgeries available at that time. It is well known that the infectious endophthalmitis that occurs after cataract surgery is usually fungal or bacterial and is often associated with intra-ocular lenses. The success of treatment varies in these cases and, while removal of the implant may be required in some situations, the implant can be retained in others with successful treatment. The general approach in surgical management of cataract extraction, with and without intra-ocular lens implantation, in uveitis patients is documented. Special problems and considerations that occur are synechiae, cyclitic membrane; inflammatory membrane over the surface of the lens, which may or may not be connected to the iris, management of the iris, vitreous cells and opacities, as well as intra-ocular lens manipulation.

At present, the indications for pars plana vitrectomy in cases of intra-ocular inflammation is twofold. It is used as a controlled biopsy of the vitreous to establish histologic diagnosis of endophthalmitis, large cell lymphoma, and other unusual infiltrations of the vitreous. But it also serves as a therapeutic intervention in many cases. A combined lensectomy-vitrectomy has recently been advocated as an intervention to ameliorate the crippling cystoid macular edema that often occurs in inflammatory diseases of the back of the eye.

Certain forms of ocular inflammation do lend themselves to diagnostic vitrectomy. This is a standard consideration for patients with large cell lymphoma (reticulum cell sarcoma), and diagnostic as well as therapeutic vitrectomy is now advocated for almost all types of endophthalmitis with the possible exclusion of *Staphylococcus aureus* and *Staphylococcus epidermidis,* which may be controlled medically. Vitrectomy has also been advocated in cases of *Toxocara canis* endophthalmitis, and all patients who are drug-abusing suspects (thought to be manifesting a profound uveitis, endophthalmitis, or both) certainly should undergo therapeutic vitreous removal, if not a diagnostic vitreous biopsy. Although the approach to suspected infectious endophthalmitis is controversial, it is generally accepted that immediate aqueous and vitreous taps for culture and smears are important first steps, and that topical, subconjunctival, and parenteral antibiotics are necessary, while the role of intravitreal antibiotics is less well defined. We feel that intravitreal antibiotics are indicated in most cases of suspected bacterial endophthalmitis and that these can be injected during aqueous and vitreous paracentesis.

There is, likewise, some general agreement that if marked vitreous exudation obscures the retinal vasculature (i.e., by indirect ophthalmoscopy), therapeutic vitrectomy is indicated by that measure as well. If the retina can be easily visualized with minimal vitreous reactions, it is probably safer to treat the patient with subconjunctival, parenteral, and intravitreal antibiotics and to follow the patient closely. If the disease progresses and there is further clouding of the vitreous, we recommend immediate vitrectomy. The vitrectomy may also allow the medications that are given parenterally and topically to penetrate more deeply, because surgical intervention is known to further disrupt the blood-retinal barrier.

The possibility of the retina having a toxic reaction to medications (i.e., amphotericin) is greater during and after vitrectomy, because the medication contacts the retina more directly. Therefore, more dilute solutions of the drugs should be used during and after the vitrectomy procedure than before.

Technically, a total vitrectomy may not be necessary and a "core" vitrectomy will suffice. The inflammatory membranes that result from endophthalmitis often adhere tightly to the retina, and a total vitrectomy can pose the threat of severely damaging the retina, although it may be necessary to peel these membranes during vitrectomy. We currently consider the indications for lensectomy-vitrectomy in patients with intra-ocular inflammation to be: (1) a need for better vision, (2) progressive disease (hypotony, premonitory signs of phthisis, especially in the presence of cyclitic membrane), (3) complications requiring surgery (e.g., retinal detachment, tractional or rhegmatogenous) and, (4) iris bombé (closed angle with synechiae) with hypotony (indicating the presence of a cyclitic membrane). A whole discussion of the technicalities of the assessment of visual functions in patients before surgery is included so that patients do not undergo surgery unnecessarily when the common end goal of vision is what is ultimately to be considered. The complications of vitrectomy (especially too aggressive a vitrectomy in certain inflammatory situations) are discussed. These complications often include retinal tears which, combined with the underlying inflammatory disorder, may eventuate in proliferative vitreoretinopathy (PVR or MPP) with subretinal membrane growth. Further, a separate chapter on endophthalmitis is included that details the recognition, the diagnosis, and the surgical techniques involved. It encompasses very specific indications for surgery, alluded to in the chapters preceding it on vitrectomy and inflammatory diseases.

A problem that goes hand in hand with the foregoing topics and presents an ever-increasing national health hazard is drug abuse. An entire chapter is dedicated to a discussion of drug abuse, the various substances that are abused, the ophthalmalogic clinical pictures that present with drug abuse, as well as the treatment of drug abuse endophthalmitis, which involves bacterial and fungal endophthalmitis. All of us as ophthalmologists must be able to recognize these complicated patients when they present. They frequently present with a myriad of strange and perplexing signs and symptoms for which the earliest intervention may prevent the most disastrous outcome. There is often needless delay because patients who are drug-abuse victims do not come forth with proper history; therefore, untoward complications (such as disastrous endophthalmitis and inflammatory retinal detachment) occur which might have been prevented with early medical or surgical intervention. Furthermore, it behooves us to try to direct these difficult patients to the appropriate physical and psychosocial health workers who will help them with the overall scope of their problem. Drug abuse ushers in a host of new considerations in the medical management of these young patients with mysterious complaints and illnesses and often a disastrous disease spectrum. A young person who has not undergone ocular surgery and who presents with what appears to be a metastatic endophthalmitis should be suspected of intravenous drug abuse until proven otherwise. These patients may also be at risk for acquired immune deficiency syndrome (AIDS) and all of the opportunistic infections that are currently killing young people. The virulence of the HIV agent causing AIDS in parenteral drug abusers is possibly related to the synergistic effect of antigenic overload from chronic exposure to chemical contamination with illicit drugs. It must also be remembered that many female drug abusers are also involved in prostitution and, increasingly, are contributing to the contagion of AIDS.

Inflammatory retinal detachment presents a great clinical challenge to the ophthalmologist. Uveitis and retinal detachment can be related in three ways: exudative retinal detachment can be a component of the underlying uveitis; uveitis can be a late complication of chronic rhegmatogenous retinal detachment; and rhegmatogenous or traction retinal detachment can be a complication of uveitis. Patients with uveitis and retinal detachment have all the clinical signs and symptoms of both disorders. Previously, retinal detachment surgery was notoriously unsuccessful in patients with underlying or secondary uveitis. The treatment of retinal detachment has progressed remarkably with the advent of vitrectomy as a coexisting procedure to help in its management. The use of air, gas, and viscous bubbles (i.e., silicon) has also helped in the surgical manipulation of the retina, and now far fewer patients with inflammatory retinal detachment experience the disastrous and untoward eventuality of progressive vitreoretinopathy (PVR, MPP).

Certain infectious etiologies, such as toxoplasmosis and *Toxocara canis*, lead to rhegmatogenous retinal detachment. These will be covered in detail. A discussion of the natural history and progression of pars planitis is included. This disorder warrants special mention as a phenomenon with continuous low-grade inflammation and often a progressive, long-term retinal traction followed by detachment. Although this occurs only in a minority of patients, it should be remembered that if they are left with none of the serious sequelae of the disease at the time of their "burn out" (i.e., cataract, glaucoma, or, most importantly, a sclerotic type of cystoid macular edema, and retinal traction or detachment), they may possess good vision for the future. One must be constantly prepared for the development of any of these complications so that intervention may allow these patients to preserve good vision with few complications.

The inception of intra-ocular inflammation in pars planitis patients is either silent or accompanied by minimal symptoms of blurred vision or floaters. By the time the condition is diagnosed, however, serious visual loss may be present in almost one half of cases. The course of pars planitis, as noted, is quite variable. In severe cases, which are rare, the perivasculitis in the posterior pole may be a prominent feature and all the retinal blood vessels, including the arteries in the retinal periphery, may close. The more usual, very benign form of pars planitis is usually slowly progressive, with many remissions and exacerbations, and becomes quiescent at an early stage. However, one must remember that the original data put forth by Schepens shows that 40% of cases of pars planitis exhibit some degree of rhegmatogenous retinal detachment, and this may occur bilaterally.

A discussion is also included on intra-ocular foreign body with uveitis, retinal detachment, or both because foreign bodies may often be a masquerade syndrome for uveitis with retinal detachment. The presence of a foreign body may be relatively infrequent in fresh cases of retinal detachment, but in cases of patients with smoldering uveitis, eyes may have harbored a foreign body for months, sometimes years, and these cases are often refractory to the usual treatment of both intra-ocular inflammation and retinal detachment. In all cases of intra-ocular foreign body there is always the danger of subsequent retinal detachment, whether it occurs at the initial injury or not.

Two metals are exceptionally toxic to the eye: iron and copper. Since the signs that these metals elicit inside the eye are pathognomonic for their damage to ocular structures, it is imperative that steps be taken for their retrieval when these signs are present, even in the absence of a positive history of ocular trauma with foreign body entrance or the localization or identification of an intra-ocular foreign body. The profound nature of the ocular disturbance depends upon the concentration of the iron or copper content of the foreign body and its location. All haste must be used to retrieve such foreign bodies as part of surgical intervention. Chalcosis, caused by copper or copper alloys, may often produce an equally violent reaction in the eye. Copper may, in fact, be the most injurious metal to the eye. When it is present in the vitreous cavity, dense infiltrates, which usually occur within just a few days of injury, adhere to the retina. Bluish-green rings form in the cornea in or near the periphery of Descemet's membrane and represent a traumatic Kayser-Fleisher ring. A sunflower cataract may be produced early, which is said to be pathognomonic of chalcosis, and the iris itself may become green with fine metallic particles visible on its surface and in the aqueous overlying it. Eyes that are subject to such metallic foreign bodies often have intractable intra-ocular inflammation until the foreign body itself is removed as part of the treatment. A concomitant rhegmatogenous detachment cannot be repaired until the foreign body is removed because of the violent exudative reaction it causes. Methods of extraction of a foreign body are detailed in a later chapter in the book.

Finally, with the advent of light energy in the treatment of various ocular disorders, a chapter on laser surgery for ocular inflammatory disease is included. This details the basic mechanism of laser use and treatment and explains the specific indications for laser treatment of ocular inflammatory disease. Adhesions and synechiae are becoming increasingly amenable to careful and detailed laser treatment of posterior capsular overgrowth in patients who have undergone extracapsular surgery with uveitis necessitating YAG laser capsulotomy. The use of laser for treatment of inflammatory vitreal bands causing traction on the retina is another frontier in the future of uveitis treatment. This application is yet one more manifestation of the laser providing the ophthalmologist with a quiet and noninvasive "knife" that can cut membranes, adhesions, and synechiae thus obviating the opening of the eye for a surgical procedure.

Surgical decisions for uveitis patients must be based upon an accurate anticipation and prediction of the added risks presented by the uveitis patient. Uveitis, as already noted, is not one disease but a collection of many different diseases linked because they all produce intra ocular inflammation. For most of the common uveitic syndromes, the course, complications, treatment, as well as short- and long-term outlook, are all quite well known. Yet, it is common to hear surgeons refer to much of uveitis as "idiopathic." By using recently described, relatively simple techniques, at least 80% of these patients can be categorized and properly placed into one of the known, common uveitic syndromes.

Approach to the Uveitis Syndrome

The basic approach needed to establish the uveitis syndrome diagnosis for these patients involves the Naming-Meshing System. This is a five-step approach that organizes the data obtained from the history and physical examination to maximize the physician's ability to arrive at the correct uveitic diagnosis.

The five steps to the Naming-Meshing System are

Naming
Meshing
Preliminary differential diagnosis
Tests, procedures, and consultations
Final uveitic diagnosis

While a complete discussion of the Naming-Meshing System is beyond the scope of this book, it has been described in detail elsewhere.* However, a brief explanation of this method, its steps, and its operation will be given here.

Naming

An accurate uveitis-directed history and physical examination of the uveitis patient can provide the greatest amount of information necessary to make the proper uveitic diagnosis. From the ocular history, if the patient has attacks of severe pain, redness, and photophobia, we can confidently conclude that he has had attacks of acute iridocyclitis. No other type of uveitis will produce symptomatology that severe. Similarly, chronic iridocyclitis will cause primarily hazy vision. Intermediate uveitis causes blurred vision and floating black spots. Posterior uveitis, without macular involvement, will cause visual haze and floating black spots if the inflammation is primarily in the retina and vitreous, and minimal or no visual symptoms when it is primarily peripheral choroiditis. Of course, if the macula is involved, then poor vision and central scotomata may be noted.

Information from the nonocular history may also produce important diagnostic information. If the patient with attacks of ocular pain, redness, and photophobia is a white male with low back pain and a positive family history of back pain or enterocolitis, this is consistent with the HLA-B27–related iridocyclitis associated with ankylosing spondylitis, Reiter's syndrome, and inflammatory bowel disease. Similarly, if the patient has attacks of pain, redness, and photophobia in either or both eyes; is a male from one of the Eastern Mediterranean

* Smith RE, Nozik RA: *Uveitis: A Clinical Approach to Diagnosis and Management.* Baltimore, Williams & Wilkins, 1983

countries; has ulcers of the mouth, tongue, and genitalia, as well as a persistent, recurrent tender rash, the diagnosis may well be Behcet's syndrome.

A properly performed, uveitis-directed physical examination of the eyes can provide information that is very useful for the establishment of the uveitic diagnosis. Information of great value will be evidence of unilaterality or bilaterality and whether the uveitis is primarily anterior, intermediate, posterior, or diffuse; granulomatous or nongranulomatous; acute, recurrent, or chronic, exacerbating or remitting. Is there retinal vasculitis? If so, is it primary or secondary, posterior or peripheral? Is there periphlebitis, arteritis, or both? Does the patient have primary retinitis and retinochoroiditis or primary choroiditis and chorioretinitis? If retinitis or choroiditis, is it focal, multifocal, disseminated, or diffuse? A careful, precise examination by the ophthalmologist can almost always provide this very important information which is necessary to achieve the "naming" or first step in the diagnostic process.

Some examples of "naming" will follow. It is important to note that all of the data in the names have accrued from the history and physical examination.

> **Example 1:** L. C. is a 38-year-old white male, who has had five attacks of pain, redness, and photophobia starting 6 years ago and never in both eyes simultaneously. He now has acute, severe, nongranulomatous iridocyclitis of the right eye and low intraocular pressure. Twelve years ago he experienced an episode of nonspecific urethritis while in the army. He has arthritis of the left knee and ankle, and he has a grandfather with chronic low back pain and a grandmother with colitis.

> **Example 2:** A 9-year-old white female with chronic, bilaterally active, nongranulomatous iridocyclitis with band keratopathy, foreshortened mandible, and chronic arthritis of the left wrist and elbow.

> **Example 3:** A 25-year-old black female with chronic, bilaterally active, low-grade granulomatous iridocyclitis with chronic cystoid macular edema of the right eye and posterior retinal periphlebitis bilaterally; intermittent, low-grade fevers of unknown origin; and intermittent pain, swelling, and redness of the fingers.

Although at first these "names" may seem to be awkward and lengthy, they are, in fact, the most economical and useful way to combine most of the important information necessary to establish the uveitic diagnosis.

Meshing

The meshing step may be thought of as comparing the unknown (the patient with uveitis) with a group of knowns (the uveitic entities; Table 1-1). Since the clinical characteristics of the 20 or 30 most common uveitic syndromes are quite well known, it is not difficult to perform this comparison. Fortunately, most of the uveitic entities present a consistent and distinctive clinical picture and are rather

(*Text continues on p. 21.*)

TABLE 1-1. Twenty-two Likely Uveitic Entities

Uveitic Entity	Anatomical*	Chronology†	Nongranulomatous (NG)#	Male-M Female-F	Unilateral-U Bilateral-B	Laboratory§	Therapy	Complications	Prognosis
Viral/nonspecific/ trauma	I	A	NG	—	U	Diagnosis based on antecedent history	Depending on severity, simple observation, mydriatic cycloplegic only, or rarely local steroids	Usually none	Good; rare recurrence
Rheumatoid spondylitis (ankylosing, psoriatic)	I-Cy	A-R	NG	M	B	ESR, HLA-B27 S-I Jt x-ray Rh Consult	Intensive local steroids (at least every 2 hrs) in attacks May need periocular and even short course high dose systemic steroids in severe cases for acute attacks No Rx between attacks unless case is converted to chronic iridocyclitis due to inadequate treatment of acute attacks—then treat as chronic nongranulomatous iridocyclitis (See juvenile rheumatoid arthritis if chronic)	Maybe none if acute attacks are treated promptly and vigorously Cataracts, posterior synechiae, glaucoma, rarely phthisis	Good if attacks are treated vigorously and promptly Poor if case is allowed to become chronic

(continued)

TABLE 1-1. Twenty-two Likely Uveitic Entities (*Continued*)

Uveitic Entity	Anatomical*	Chronology†	Nongranulomatous (NG)#	Male-M Female-F	Unilateral-U Bilateral-B	Laboratory§	Therapy	Complications	Prognosis
Reiter's syndrome	I-Cy	A-R	NG	M	B	ESR, HLA B-27 S-I Jt x-ray Med consult (chlamydial CF, cult)	Same as rheumatoid spondylitis	Same as rheumatoid spondylitis	Same as rheumatoid spondylitis
Immunologic (altered iris vascular permeability, focus of infection, immunogenic focus)	I-Cy	A-R, C	NG	—	U	Search for systemic focus, ESR Med consult	Same as rheumatoid spondylitis, but there is greater danger of converting to a chronic nongranulomatous iridocyclitis (see juvenile rheumatoid arthritis if chronic)	Same as rheumatoid spondylitis	Same as rheumatoid spondylitis; if chronic, see juvenile rheumatoid arthritis
Juvenile rheumatoid arthritis, uveitis in young girls	I-Cy	C	NG	F	B	ESR, ANA Ped consult	Use medium strength mydriatic/cycloplegic agent at least night-time even in remissions Intensive (at least every 2 hr) steroids and more frequent mydriatic cycloplegic during exacerbations	Posterior synechiae, secluded pupil, pupillary block glaucoma, secondary glaucoma, cataract, band	Very poor even with close follow-up, especially for pauciarticular cases Pts. handle intraocular surgery very poorly Due to extreme danger of

							May need periocular or systemic steroids during exacerbations Some pts. do well on low dose chronic systemic steroids	keratopathy, severe danger of ultimate phthisis	ultimate phthisis, avoid glaucoma surgery if at all possible
Heterochromic iridocyclitis	Cy, I-Cy	C	NG	—	U	—	No treatment needed in vast majority of cases Night-time dilatation with short acting mydriatic cycloplegic agents only if Koeppe nodules are present Periocular steroids for posterior polar edema (very rare)	Cataract Glaucoma	Good with no treatment Do well with cataract surgery
Chronic cyclitis/ peripheral uveitis/pars planitis	Cy	C	NG	—	B	Fluorescein	Periocular (posterior sub Tenons) repository steroids for secondary macular or disc edema only Occasional short course systemic steroids for exacerbations or immunosuppressive agents or cyclocryotherapy may be considered for severe recalcitrant cases	Macular cystoid and cyst formation Cataract, secondary steroid glaucoma	Good if cases are treated vigorously for systemic macular edema Cases do well with cataract surgery

(*continued*)

TABLE 1-1. Twenty-two Likely Uveitic Entities (*Continued*)

Uveitic Entity	Anatomical*	Chronology†	Nongranulomatous (NG)#	Male-M Female-F	Unilateral-U Bilateral-B	Laboratory§	Therapy	Complications	Prognosis
Toxocara	Cy/ macular/ End	C	G/ng‡	—	U	ELISA test for toxocara (vitreous aspiration) ESR, CBC, EOS (AC tap for EOS) (B-scan for calcification) (Ocular x-ray dental film for calcification)	Periocular steroids and/or systemic steroids during active period	Cataract, macular scar, glaucoma, retinal detachment	If macula is involved, prognosis is poor If endophthalmitis is present, prognosis is poor If involvement is peripheral, prognosis is good with treatment of severe phases of inflammation Once case is quiet for an extended period, intraocular surgery is tolerated well
Toxoplasma	R, R-Ch	A-R	G	—	—	Toxoplasma dye or FA test or ELISA test for toxoplasmosis	Vigorous treatment for lesions of macula, maculapapillary bundle, optic nerve, severe	Secondary anterior uveitis with posterior synechiae, secondary	Good if active lesion(s) is away from macula or optic nerve Fair to poor if

							endophthalmic, and macular edema secondary to lesions superior to the macula Standard treatment: Daraprim and sulfa, can use sulfa alone, can use tetracycline, and can use systemic or periocular clindamycin Concurrent systemic steroids may be of benefit Avoid periocular steroids Avoid systemic steroids without antimicrobial coverage	glaucoma, secondary cataract Retinal scarring Detached retina	lesion is in or near macula Recurrences are common and posterior, macular threatening lesions may recur over and over, eventually affecting the foveal region
Cytomegalic inclusion	R, R-Ch	A-R	G	—	B	Virus studies of urine, serum (tears) Ped consult, CF test	Same as toxoplasma, however no antimicrobial agents are available, so moderate systemic steroids may be necessary in macular threatening lesions without	Same as toxoplasma	Same as toxoplasma

(*continued*)

TABLE 1-1. Twenty-two Likely Uveitic Entities (*Continued*)

Uveitic Entity	Anatomical*	Chronology†	Nongranulomatous (NG)#	Male-M Female-F	Unilateral-U Bilateral-B	Laboratory§	Therapy	Complications	Prognosis
							antimicrobial coverage High doses of systemic steroids and immunosuppressive drugs are contraindicated, and may in fact, cause exacerbation Transfer factor as well as adenine arabinoside may be helpful		
Birdshot	R-Ch, RPE, RV, (I-Cy)	C	NG	—	B	Fluorescein	Systemic and/or periocular steroids (often poor result)	Cystoid/cystic macular edema and scarring	Fair to poor
Acute multifocal posterior placoid epitheliopathy	RPE, I-Cy	A	NG	—	B	Fluorescein (R/o systemic virus infection)	—	Macular pigment alteration and scarring	Fair to poor
Geographic choroiditis Serpiginous choroidopathy	Ch, RPE, (I-Cy)	A-R	NG	—	B	Fluorescein	—	Macular scarring	Fair to poor (good if macula spared)

Helicoid choroidopathy									
Histoplasma	Ch	A-R	G	—	B	Histoplasma skin test Chest x-ray HLA B-7	Vigorous treatment of symptoms of metamorphopsia with high dose short course systemic steroids may be helpful Periocular steroids may help Photocoagulation of macula threatening lesions may be of benefit	Macular scarring	Good if no lesion is in macula Fair to poor if lesion (even fluorescein window defect) is present in macula due to recurrent activity and ultimate development of subretinal neovascular net
Tuberculosis	I-Cy, Cy, Ch, RV	C, A-R	G	—	B	Tbc skin test, chest x-ray, ESR Med consult (serum lysozyme)	Treat acute recurrent iridocyclitis as in rheumatoid spondylitis Treat chronic iridocyclitis as in juvenile rheumatoid arthritis Treat active choroiditis lesions with systemic steroids covered by antituberculosis therapy (INH)	Cataract, glaucoma, macula and optic nerve scarring, phthisis	Mixed depending on character of individual case and especially related to chronicity of inflammatory activity Cataract surgery is fairly well tolerated in cases which have been quiet for a long term Poorly tolerated in cases which are chronically active

(*continued*)

TABLE 1-1. Twenty-two Likely Uveitic Entities (*Continued*)

Uveitic Entity	Anatomical*	Chronology†	Nongranulomatous (NG)#	Male-M Female-F	Unilateral-U Bilateral-B	Laboratory§	Therapy	Complications	Prognosis
Sarcoid	I-Cy, Cy, RV	C-R	G/ng	—	B	Chest x-ray, skin test anergy to Tbc, mumps, etc.; conj. biopsy, Schirmer, ESR Med consult ACE (serum lysozyme) Gallium scan, (serum proteins) (serum Ca, PO_4) (x-ray hands and feet) (Kveim)	Same as tuberculosis but no antituberculosis therapy necessary	Same as tuberculosis	Same as tuberculosis
Behçet	I-Cy, R-Ch, RV	A-R, C	NG/G	M	B	Med consult fluorescein (skin puncture test) HLA-B5, Behçet's antibody test	Intensive local and/or systemic steroids for acute exacerbations Periocular steroids for acute exacerbations	Same as toxoplasma	Same as toxoplasma

							May need low dose chronic local or systemic steroid use in chronic cases Immunosuppressive agents (esp. cyclosporine chlorambucil) are often very effective in difficult cases (colchicine)		
Vogt-Koyanagi-Harada	I-Cy, Ch-R, Ch	A-R, C	NG/G	—	B	LP during attacks, fluorescein, Med consult Skin and hair follicle biopsy for absence of melanocytes HLA-BW22J HLA-LDWa	Same as Behçet	Same as tuberculosis	Same as tuberculosis
Sympathetic Ophthalmia	I-Cy, Ch	C	NG/G	M	B	—	Same as Behçet	Same as tuberculosis	Same as tuberculosis
Luetic	Anything	A-R, C	G/ng***	—	B	VDRL, FTA Abs Med consult	Same as tuberculosis; however, instead of antituberculosis therapy use antiluetic therapy	Same as tuberculosis	Same as tuberculosis
Fungal endophthalmitis	End, R	A, A-R, C	G/ng	M	U, B	Biopsy active area (especially vitreous)	Amphotericin B (systemic intravitreal), flucytosine	Persistent uveitis, retinal detachment, phthisis	Generally poor with some exceptions

(*continued*)

TABLE 1-1. Twenty-two Likely Uveitic Entities (*Continued*)

Uveitic Entity	Anatomical*	Chronology†	Nongranulomatous (NG)#	Male-M Female-F	Unilateral-U Bilateral-B	Laboratory§	Therapy	Complications	Prognosis
Reticulum cell sarcoma (B-cell lymphoma)	I-Cy, vitritis subretinal infiltrate	C	G/ng	—	U, B	Vitreous biopsy, immunologic stain of light chains Med consult CT scan brain LP	Chemo Rx, radiation	Usually lethal	Generally prognosis poor

* I, Iritis; I-Cy, iridocyclitis; Cy, cyclitis; R, retinitis; Ch, choroiditis; R-Ch, retinochoroiditis; Ch-R, chorioretinitis; End, endophthalmitis; RV, retinal vasculitis; RPE, inflammation of retinal pigment epithelium
† A, acute; A-R, acute-recurrent; C, chronic
‡ If lowercase, this is of lesser importance.
§ Laboratory Abbreviations

ACE	Angiotensin converting enzyme
ANA	Antinuclear antibodies
Ca	Calcium
CBC	Complete blood count
CF	Complement fixation
Cult	Culture
ELISA	Enzyme-linked immunosorbent assay
EOS	Eosinophil count
ESR	Erythrocyte sedimentation rate
FA	Fluorescent antibody test
FTA-Abs	Fluorescent treponemal antibody absorption test
HLA	Human leukocyte antigen
LP	Lumbar puncture
Med consult	Medical consultation
Ped consult	Pediatric consultation
PO_4	Phosphate radical
Rh consult	Rheumatologic consultation
S-I Jt x-ray	Sacroiliac joint x-ray
Tbc	Tuberculosis
VDRL	Venereal disease research laboratory test

Laboratory tests in parentheses are those of lesser importance.

easily separated, one from the others. It is, of course, necessary for the ophthalmologist using this system to become familiar with the major clinical characteristics of the various common uveitic syndromes in order to use the meshing step properly. In using the meshing step, usually one will find only two, three, or at most four different uveitic entities that will be similar enough to the unknown, the patient, to be included in a preliminary differential diagnostic list.

Preliminary Differential Diagnosis

This step is the result generated from the meshing step. One need only evaluate how good the fit is between the specific uveitic patient and each of the uveitic entities generated in the meshing step. This differential diagnostic list is then ranked in descending order with the best fit listed first.

Tests, Procedures, and Consultations

This step represents a fine-tuning of the diagnostic process. For each of the uveitic entities, starting with the most likely, various tests may be ordered. Exactly which tests and consultations to order may be obtained from any standard reference.* These results may then be used to effect a final reordering of the differential diagnostic list. Table 1-1 provides a complete listing of diagnostic considerations for uveitis.

Final Uveitic Diagnosis

The modification applied to the preliminary differential diagnostic list will yield the final uveitic diagnosis in over 80% of uveitic cases seen by the general ophthalmologist.

The course, proper treatment, complications, and long-term prognosis are known for each of the common uveitic entities. Therefore, once the uveitic diagnosis has been determined, the decisions regarding whether or not to operate, which operation to use, or how to modify the surgery to best suit the case can be made rationally and in a way to best effect a favorable outcome.

In order to be successful when operating on uveitis patients, the ophthalmic surgeon must go beyond the diagnosis of idiopathic uveitis in the majority of cases.

* Smith RE, Nozik RA: *Uveitis: A Clinical Approach to Diagnosis and Management.* Baltimore, Williams & Wilkins, 1983

TWO

Paracentesis of the Eye

The dazzling panorama of new diagnostic laboratory techniques allows for the identification and characterization of cells, proteins, histopathologic specimens, and even ultrastructural analysis on very small samples obtained by paracentesis. Diagnostic paracentesis of the eye (keratocentesis of the anterior chamber fluid) and vitreous biopsy (paracentesis of the vitreous fluid in the posterior segment of the eye) have definite value (1) in determining specific microbial pathogens which are the likely cause of infectious disease in the eye; (2) in identifying the predominance of certain cell types (i.e., eosinophiles, macrophages; epithelial ingrowth, "ghost erythrocytes," "phacolytic cells") which may provide a clue to the etiology of an inflammatory disease which may be autoimmune or allergic in nature; and (3) in the possible identification of specific antibodies in the aqueous humor or vitreous aspirate which would be suggestive of infection with organisms such as *Toxocara, Toxoplasma,* herpesvirus, syphilis; of other proteins such as lens proteins; or of angiotensin converting enzyme, suggestive of granulomatous inflammation such as sarcoidosis (Table 2-1). Immune complexes and antibodies associated with Behçet's disease may be found. Tumor cells may be identified when a malignant infiltration of the eye masquerades as a uveitis (large-cell lymphoma, leukemia, retinoblastoma, malignant melanoma, and other metastatic disease), as well as tumor cell enzymes and antigens.[60,69]

While keratocentesis had been advocated in a prior epoch as a treatment for active uveitis, it fell beyond the attention of the ophthalmologist until the second

TABLE 2-1. Diagnostic Paracentesis: Findings

Finding	Condition or Disease Indicated
Aqueous	
Bacteria	Endophthalmitis
Fungi	*Candida, Aspergillus,* etc.
Tumor cells	Retinoblastoma, malignant melanoma, reticulum cell sarcoma, leukemia, metastatic cancer
Eosinophils	*Toxocara canis*
Macrophages	Phakolytic glaucoma
Antibodies (ELISA)	*Toxoplasma gondii*
	Toxocara canis
	Reticulum cell sarcoma, Behçet's disease,[58] syphilis
Immune complexes	Behçet's disease
Other proteins	
Angiotensin-converting enzyme	Sarcoid
Lactate dehydrogenase isoenzymes	Retinoblastoma
Lens fragments	Phacolytic glaucoma
Ghost erythrocytes	Hemorrhagic glaucoma
Metastatic cancer cells	Metastatic cancer
JXG	JXG
Mesenchymal fibrous cells	PHPV
Amyloid	Amyloid
Epithelial cells	Epithelial ingrowth
Vitreous	
Bacteria	Endophthalmitis
Fungi	*Candida, Aspergillus* sp., etc.
Tumor cells	Retinoblastoma, malignant melanoma, reticulum cell sarcoma, leukemia, metastatic cancer
Eosinophils	*Toxocara canis*
Antibodies	*Toxoplasma gondii,* reticulum cell sarcoma, Behçet's disease,[58] syphilis (and immune complexes)
Macrophages	Sympathetic ophthalmia, severe retinitis
Amyloid	Amyloid
Calcium soaps	Asteroid hyalosis

decade of the 20th century when Bruckner first examined the aqueous humor for diagnostic purposes.[1] With the explosion in laboratory techniques to evaluate very small aliquots of fluid (i.e., 0.2–0.3 ml of aqueous or vitreous) and the ability to identify specific microbial organisms, the predominance of other cell types, antibodies, and proteins in these fluids, there has mushroomed a very specific and helpful adjunct to the diagnosis of those sight-threatening ocular inflammations that provide a diagnostic dilemma and necessitate paracentesis intervention. Witmer and O'Connor have provided strong evidence that samples of the aqueous humor reflect the antibody-producing capabilities of the iris and ciliary body, particularly when more specific antibody per unit of gamma globulin can be found on the aqueous humor than in the blood of the same patient.[2 to 5] These determinations may be highly significant when one considers the fact that diseased tissue is being bathed in an antibody-containing fluid that is elaborated locally (see Figs. 2-1, 2-2, and 2-3, where the immunofluorescent antibody titer to toxoplasmosis is four times greater in the vitreous aspirate, at time of vitrectomy for repair of retinal detachment, than in the plasma). These same considerations have long been recognized in syphilis of the central nervous system, wherein specific antibodies may be present in the cerebrospinal fluid but not in the blood. This was also the case with an unusual presentation of ocular coccidioidomycosis.[6]

Many forms of uveitis are characterized by specific types of inflammatory cells (Figs. 2-4, 2-5). Usually, however, one encounters mixtures of cell types in any given specimen, with the relative percentages of lymphocytes and polymorphonuclear cells varying. There may be unusual numbers of eosinophils (see Fig. 2-2), or the presence of macrophages laden with lens material. Thus, an enumeration of the cells and a careful analysis of their structure can be useful as a diagnostic aid. Fig. 2-2 demonstrates eosinophils that were aspirated from the anterior chamber of a patient with *Toxocara canis* endophthalmitis. Fig. 2-3

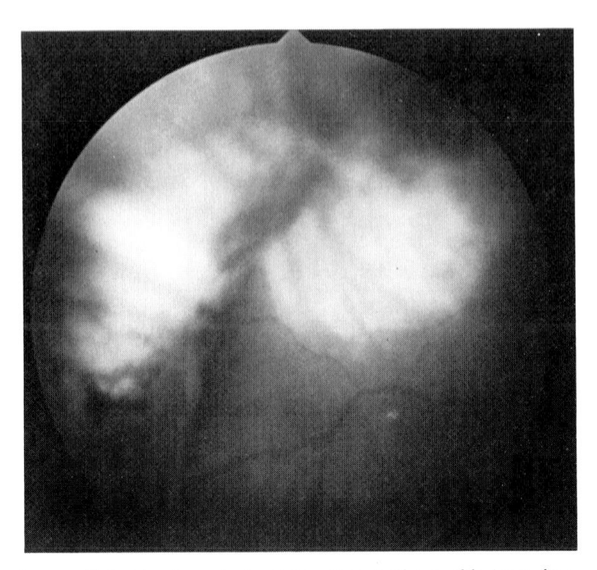

Figure 2-1. Fundus photograph of a patient with toxoplasmosis who after vitrectomy and scleral buckling, demonstrates the etiologic chorioretinal lesion at the 11:30 position on the buckle, which is now inactive. The patient's serum IFA toxoplasmosis titer was 1:1024 in the plasma; the vitrectomy fluid yielded a titer of 1:4096.

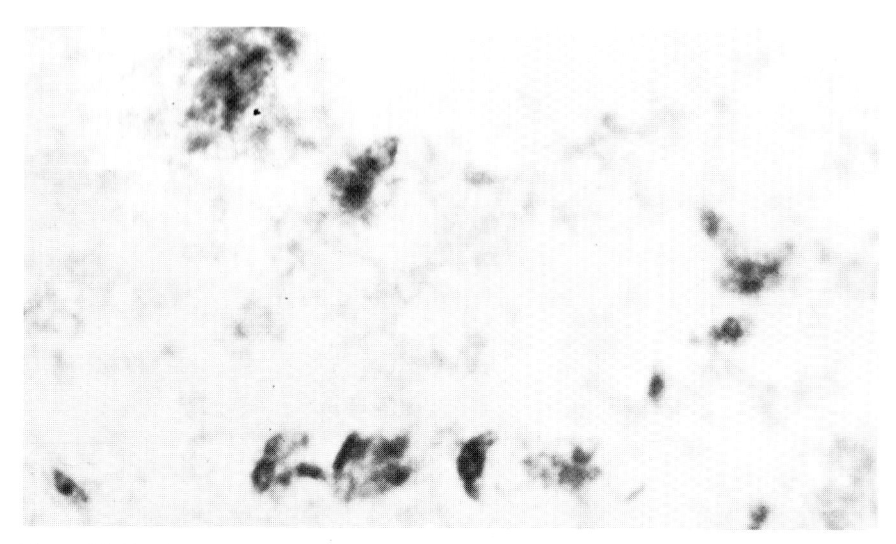

Figure 2-2. Trophozoites of toxoplasmosis on aspirate from mouse peritoneum, which incubated acute material from a patient with acute acquired systemic toxoplasmosis with retinitis.

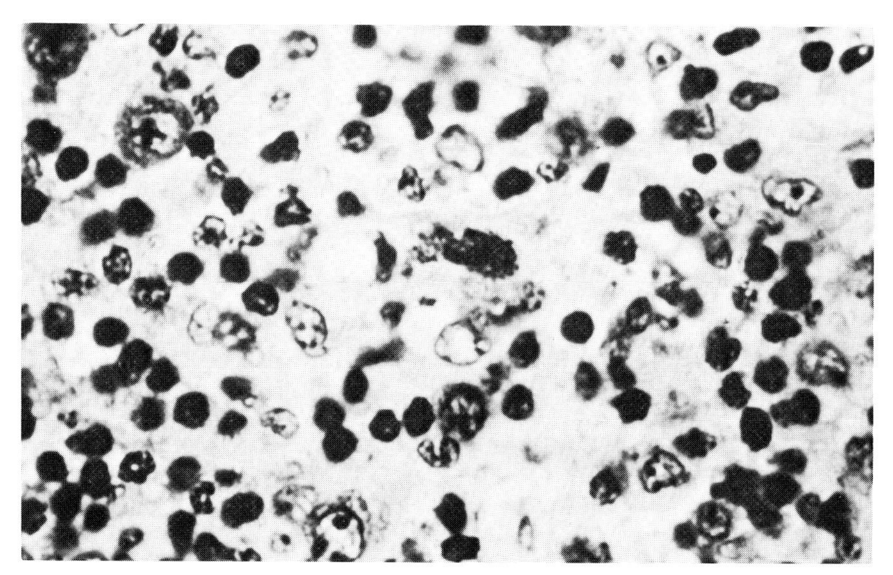

Figure 2-3. Axillary lymph node of a patient with acquired systemic toxoplasmosis demonstrates trophozoites and a toxoplasma cyst.

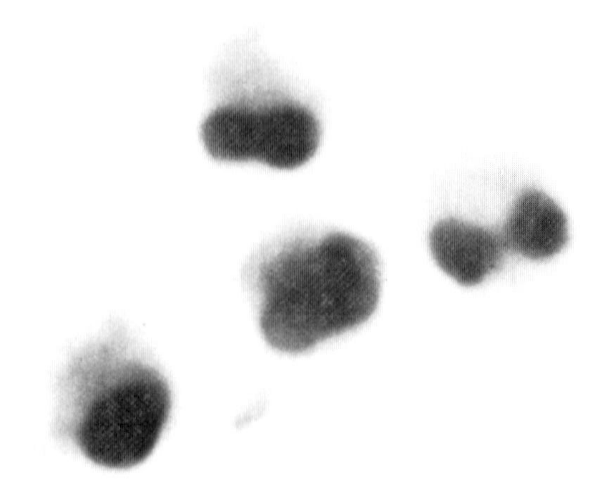

Figure 2-4. Multinucleated eosinophils in an aqueous specimen of a patient with *Toxocara canis* endophthalmitis.

demonstrates malignant cell infiltrate from the vitreous, showing the stained presence of monoclonal light chains being elaborated in the cytoplasm.

Precise identification and culture of bacterial and fungal pathogens can be obtained from both the aqueous humor and the vitreous fluid (Figs. 2-6, 2-7, 2-8, 2-9, and 2-10). Gram and Giemsa stain smears of centrifuged specimens from the

(*Text continues on p. 31.*)

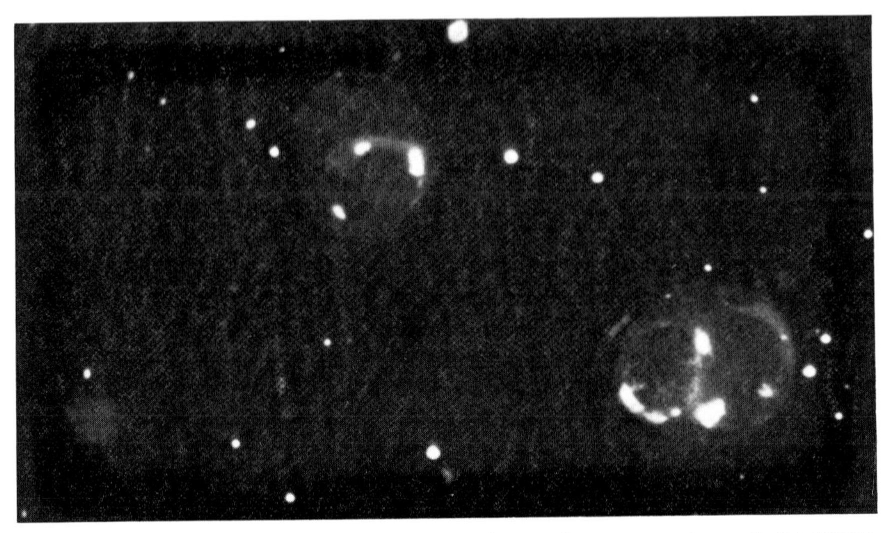

Figure 2-5. Large cell lymphoma aspirate of vitreous immunofluorescence demonstrates a monoclonal infiltrate of Lambda light chains on the B cells.

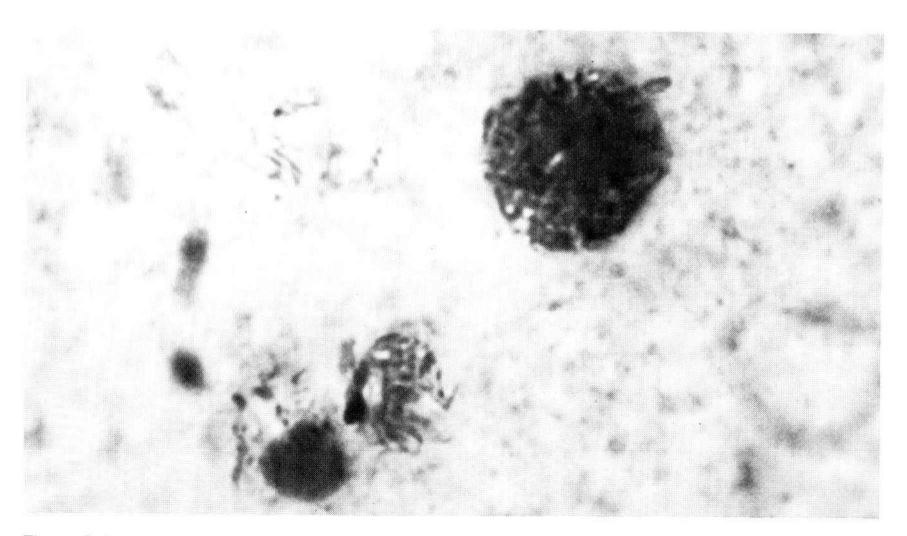

Figure 2-6. Aqueous specimen demonstrating acid-fast bacilli of acute lepromatous leprosy in the aqueous aspiration of a patient with a profound anterior segment inflammation, which presented as a diagnostic dilemma.

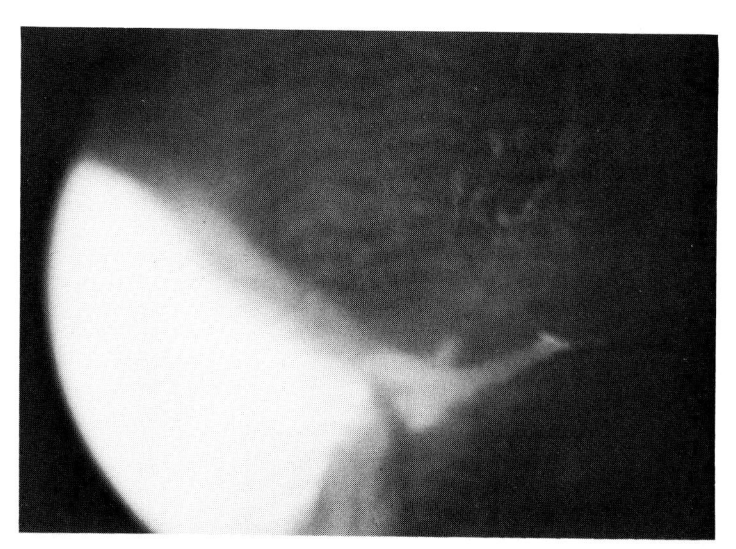

Figure 2-7. Clinical photograph of the *Toxocara* abscess in the peripheral retina with its fibrous band leading back to the posterior pole, a clinical finding thought to be pathognomonic of *Toxocara* infestation. Note the hazy vitreous inflammation obscuring much of the retinal detail below.

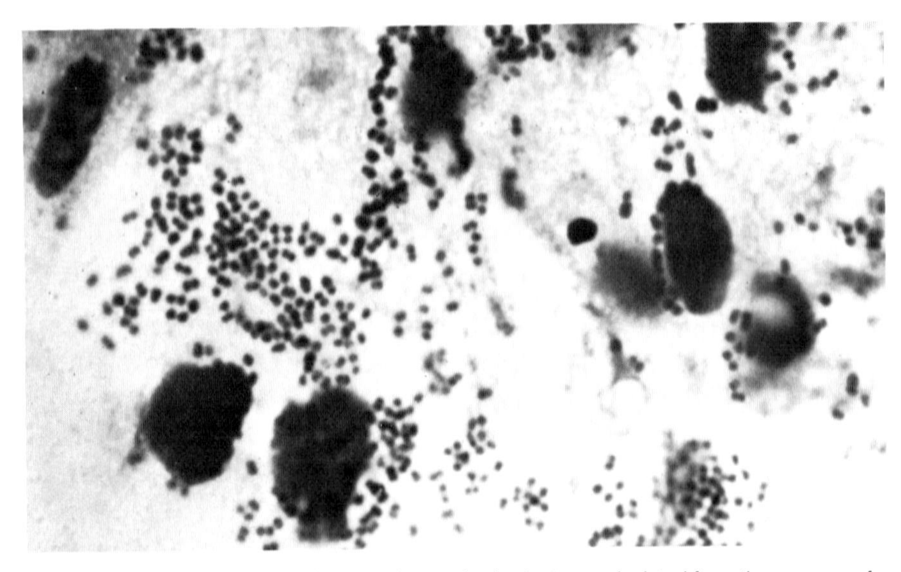

Figure 2-8. The typical gram-positive cocci occurring in clusters as isolated from the aqueous of a patient with staphylococcal endophthalmitis.

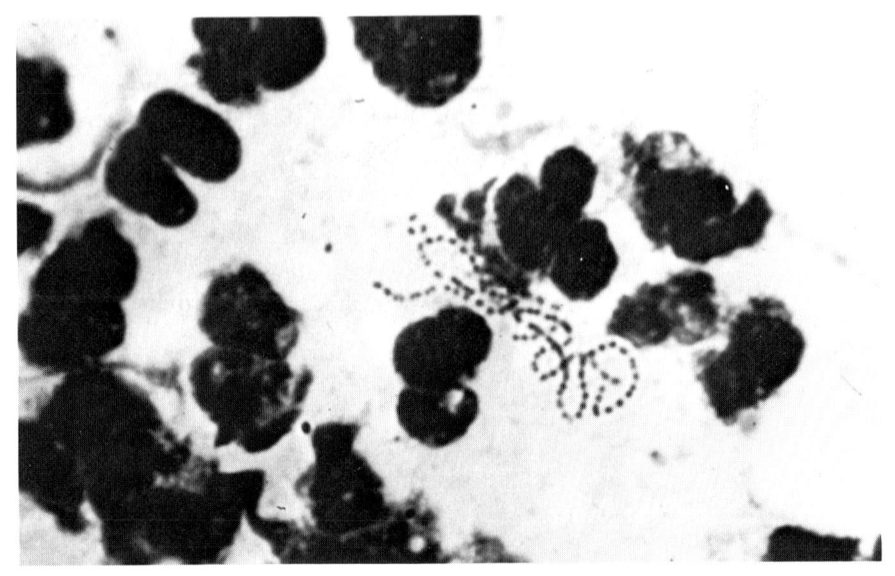

Figure 2-9. Chains of gram-positive cocci obtained from aqueous fluid in a patient with strepto-coccal endophthalmitis.

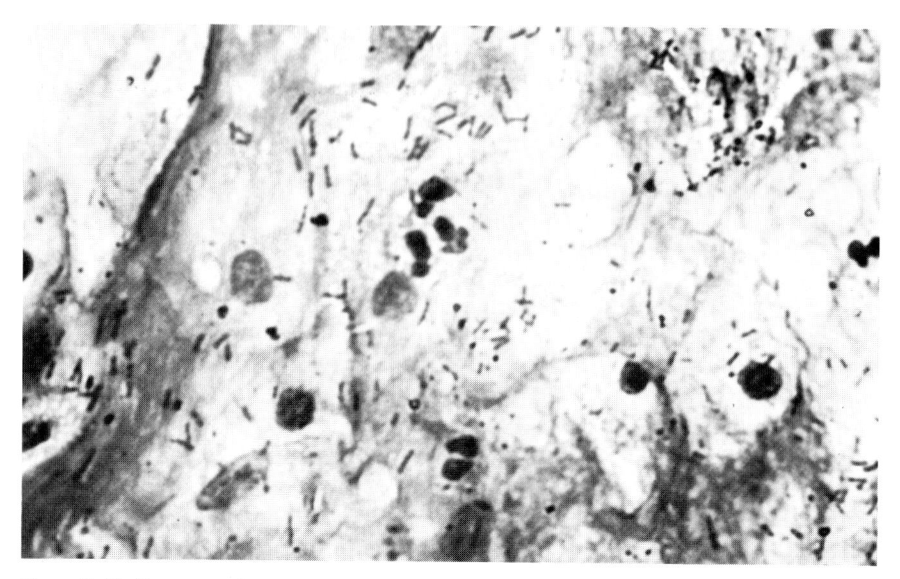

Figure 2-10. Gram-negative rods obtained from the vitreous of a patient with endophthalmitis.

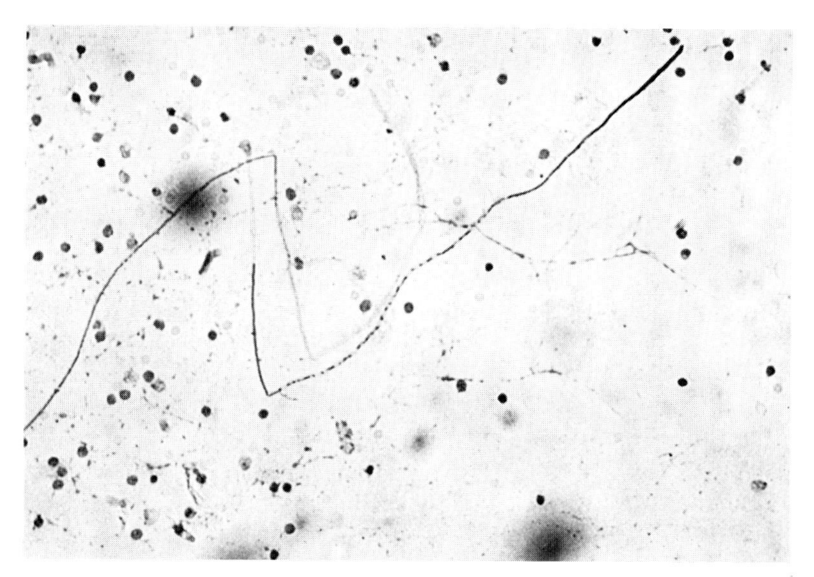

Figure 2-11. Septate hypha amid polymorphonuclear leukocytes and cellular debris of vitreous specimen isolated from a patient with *Aspergillus* endophthalmitis due to intravenous drug abuse.

aqueous humor and the vitreous humor frequently demonstrate the bacterial or fungal causative agent. Attempts to isolate bacteria and fungi and to identify them on Gram or Giemsa stain smears have been most rewarding in cases of postoperative endophthalmitis (Figs. 2-11, 2-12, 2-13, and 2-14), in cases of infection following penetrating injury of the eye, in drug-abusing patients with endogenous endophthalmitis, in patients receiving hyperalimentation, and in those patients who are immunocompromised by use of exogenous immunosuppressive agents. Allensmith, Forster, Peyman, and colleagues[7–13] have demonstrated the usefulness of ocular paracentesis for the identification of ocular infections in order to implement sight-saving treatment. Even acid-fast bacilli and viruses may be diagnosed in this fashion when emergency dictates (Figs. 2-15, 2-16, and 2-17).[14] It is recommended that diagnostic paracentesis be performed in all cases of postoperative endophthalmitis. Further, any patient over age 65 presenting with a uveitis (most usually with vitritis as the predominant infiltrate) of undetermined etiology, in which the condition of the eye is worsening, should undergo paracentesis of the vitreous to rule out reticulum cell sarcoma (large-cell lymphoma; Figs. 2-18, 2-19).[15] Any patient suspected of intravenous drug abuse who presents with an endogenous endophthalmitis or uveitis should similarly be subject to diagnostic paracentesis for fear of an intra-ocular infection being borne by the bloodstream.[16,17]

(*Text continues on p. 35.*)

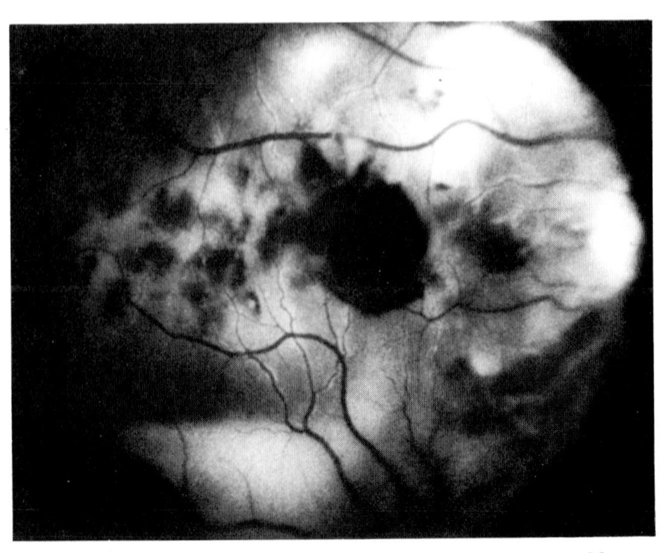

Figure 2-12. Profound retinal hemorrhage and inflammation in a 23-year-old drug abusing patient whose subretinal exudation is so dense that it formed a meniscus as its superior edge. Vitreous aspiration in this patient proved diagnostic and enabled early therapeutic intervention, which resulted in the salvaging of a useful eye.

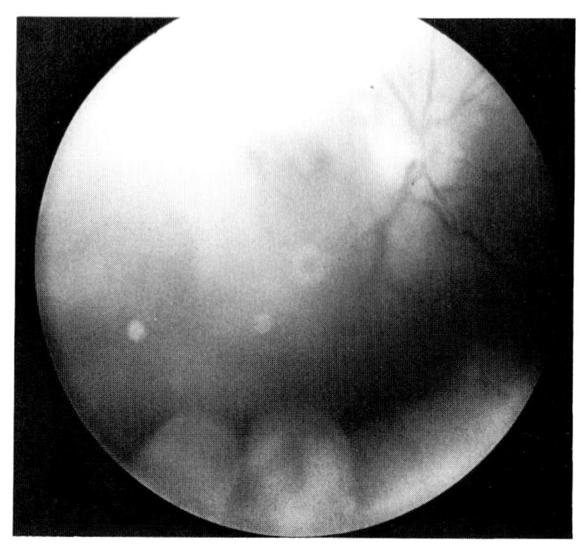

Figure 2-13. Profound intravitreal inflammation obscuring most retinal detail, except for "peek" of the optic nerve head and a small surrounding patch of retina, in a patient with *Aspergillus* endophthalmitis who underwent early vitrectomy as a consequence of retrieval of hyphae on vitreous sampling.

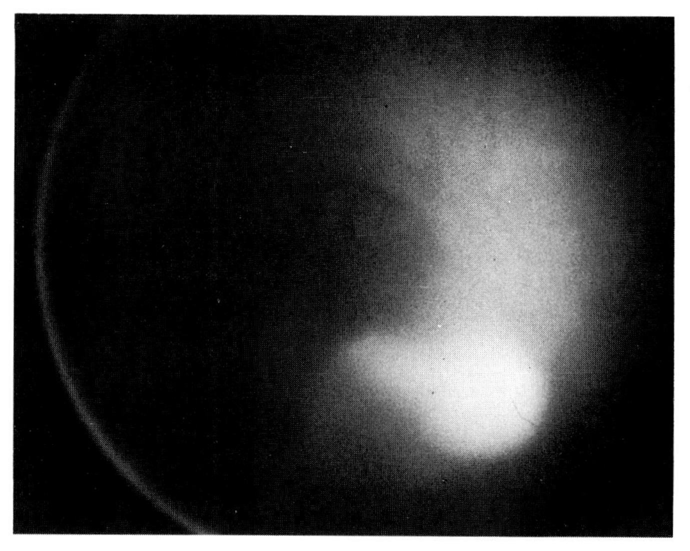

Figure 2-14. Classic presentation of *Candida* endophthalmitis demonstrating vitreous fluff balls and vitreal inflammation obscuring the retina in a 25-year-old drug abusing patient in whom *Candida albicans* was easily identified and cultured from the vitreous.

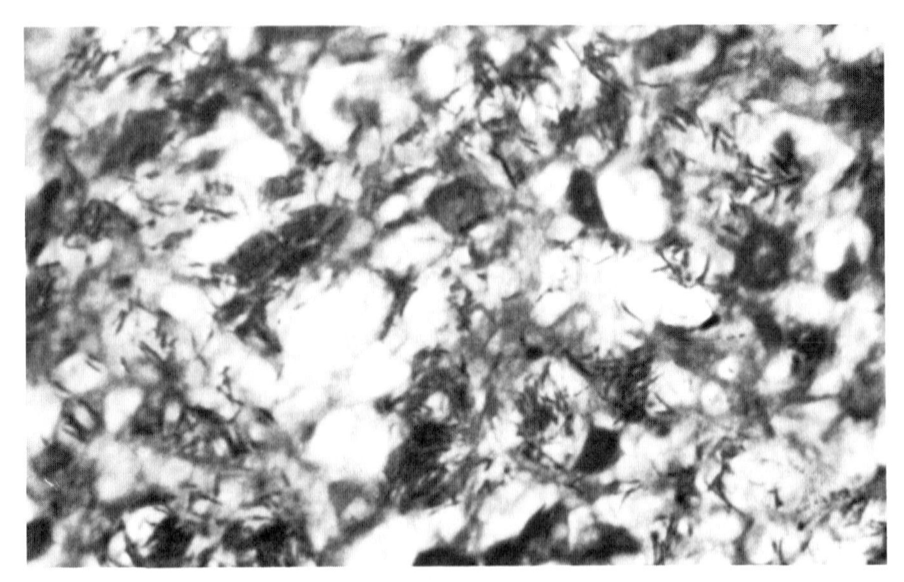

Figure 2-15. Scleral nodule showing a profuse number of acid-fast bacilli from a patient with lepromatous uveitis.

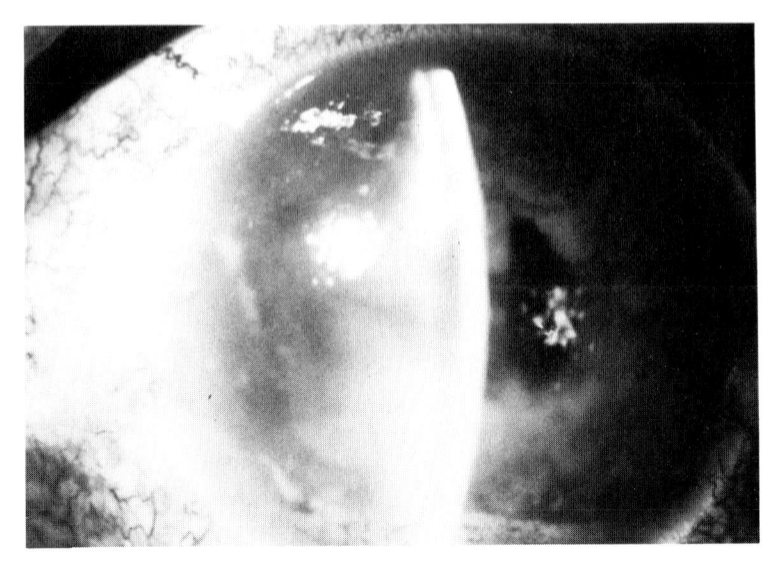

Figure 2-16. Anterior segment photograph showing petechiae-speckled hypopyon in a patient with a profound anterior segment inflammation due to acute lepromatous leprosy.

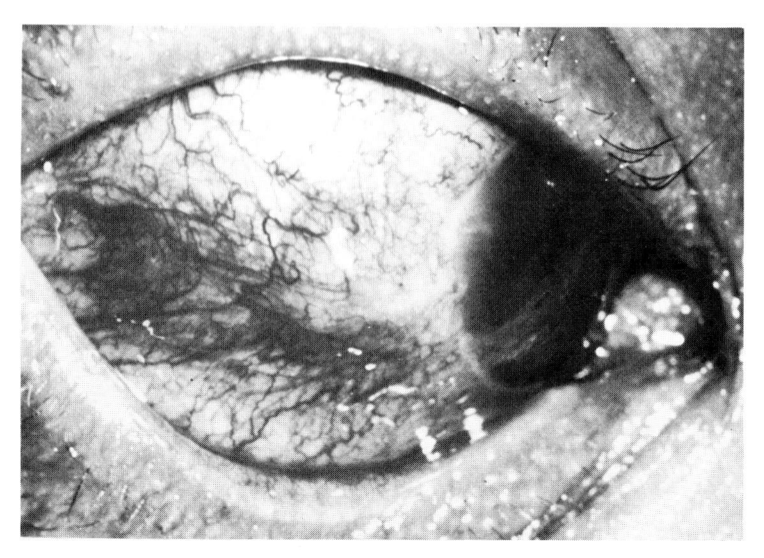

Figure 2-17. Inflamed scleral nodule removed from the same patient who had acute lepromatous uveitis.

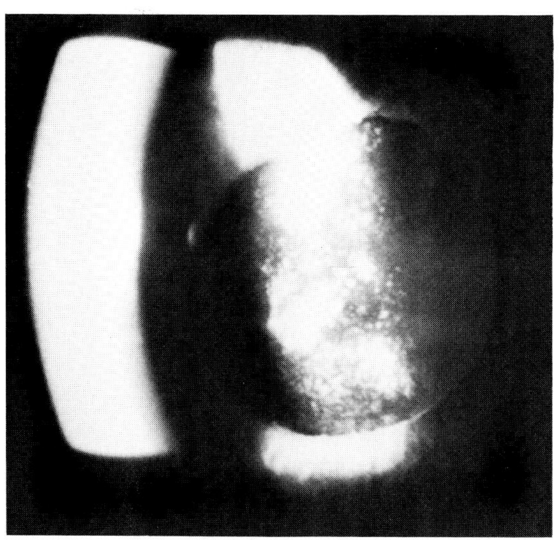

Figure 2-18. Clinical photograph showing synechiae in a patient with an exuberant aqueous infiltration of cells yielding a plastic iritis.

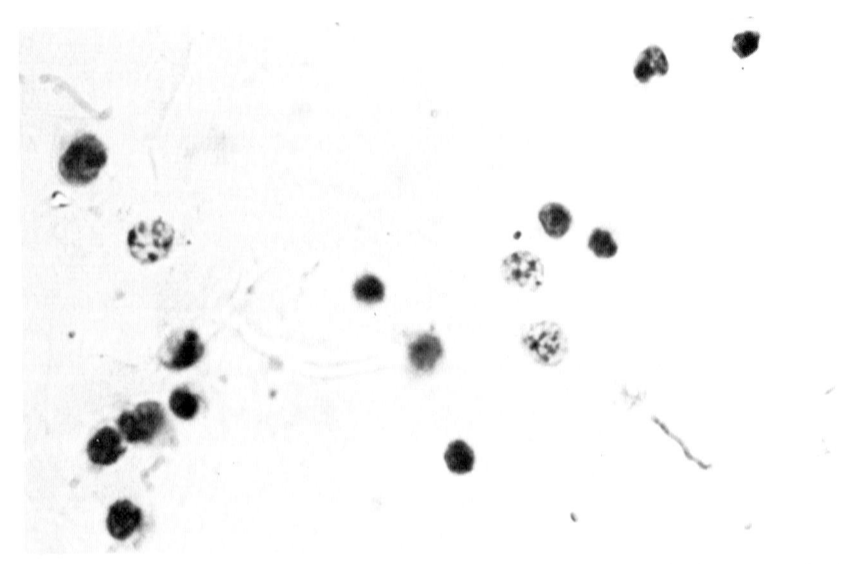

Figure 2-19. Vitreous aspirate demonstrating large cell lymphoma infiltration in a patient with vitritis and masquerade uveitis of "reticulum cell sarcoma" or large cell lymphoma.

Technique

Many techniques have been described for paracentesis of the eye. Most authorities agree that aspiration of the aqueous fluid, that is, keratocentesis, is best accomplished by the following technique: a bevelled keratotomy through peripheral clear limbal cornea is made with a Zeigler knife, a razor blade, or a super blade deeply incising the cornea but not entering the anterior chamber. A 27-gauge needle attached to a 1-ml tuberculin syringe or a 3-ml syringe is then used to enter the anterior chamber through this incision with a rolling technique. Care should be exercised to avoid touching corneal endothelium and, particularly, the lens in phakic patients. One should be careful to stay over peripheral iris at all times and should not aim the needle tip toward the center of the pupil. The yield of 0.1 to 0.3 ml of aqueous is obtained and then is immediately innoculated onto media that include blood agar, brain heart infusion, chocolate agar, and thyoglycolate liquid to be maintained at body temperature; and onto Sabouraud agar, blood agar, and brain heart infusion with gentamicin to be maintained at room temperature for fungal isolation. Care must be exercised to place the drops of aspirate away from the edges of the plate. The mouths of the tubes of the liquid media should have been flamed before use and after innoculation. Very tiny drops may be left on the tip of the syringe after innoculation of the media to prepare for Gram and Giemsa stain as well as for a methamine silver stain. Several drops per media plate may be allowed and one drop is allowed to flow several centimeters on the surface. One can roll the plate in one's finger to make sure that it has adequate coverage in the center.

In aphakic patients, a second tuberculin syringe may be fitted to a 22-gauge needle and passed through a slightly larger keratotomy incision and into the vitreous, where it may be manipulated until 0.2 to 0.3 ml of liquid vitreous aspirate is obtained. In phakic patients suspected of endophthalmitis complicating filtering bleb, trauma, or a metastatic cancer etiology, the vitreous may be aspirated through a sclerotomy at the pars plana 3.5 to 4.5 mm posterior to the limbus on the temporal side, with or without an accompanying anterior chamber paracentesis. The conjunctiva should be incised over this area down to clean sclera so that there is no obstruction when making the sclerotomy stab. If an inadequate vitreous specimen is obtained or if a fungal etiology is suspected, the pars plana incision is enlarged to 2.5 mm and a larger bore needle should be introduced to ensure that an adequate amount of liquid vitreous may be aspirated. If an infectious etiology is certain and it is suspected that a therapeutic vitrectomy will have to be undertaken in any event, it is best to do a vitreous aspiration using a vitreous suction-cutter machine, such as an Ocutome, a Peyman unit, or a Visc, which will be introduced to remove formed vitreous. It must be remembered that suction of the vitreous in a patient with endophthalmitis is very "sticky." The vitreous will have a tendency to put traction on the retina, leading to unanticipated tearing and splitting of the retina with an ultimate retinal detachment. It is best (1) to aspirate vitreous in the operating room under sterile conditions and under the controlled suction and cutting of a vitreous instrument; (2) to minimize traction on the retina from vitreous condensation and fibrous tissue formations. This is highly preferable to the unstable "sucking-only" of a large bore needle aspiration at the pars plana. The cutting rate of the vitrectomy instrument should be turned up higher than 300 cuts per minute, which will further serve to minimize tractional forces. Too much cutting of the vitreous, however, will disturb, disrupt, contort, and destroy whatever cellular elements and hyphae one may wish to obtain from the vitreous specimen. The optimum degree of vitreous surgery should include aspiration with a minimum of cutting of cellular elements but with enough rapid cutting not to prolong tractional forces. Such a vitreous sample, diluted by the irrigating solution, is then passed through a disposable membrane filter system. Adequate sterile technique must be maintained. The procedure for obtaining the vitreous would include a stop-cock assembly somewhere in the line before the machine receptacle is encountered by the sterile line. This will vary with each machine used but some forethought to the system will allow for sterile maintenance of the fluid.

Keratocentesis can be performed carefully in the office at the slit lamp with a minimum of complications. The same manipulative criteria must be observed—that is to avoid the corneal endothelium and to avoid rupturing anterior lens capsule in phakic patients. Although the conditions for vitreous aspiration would indicate the absolute sterility of the operating room and the more optimal aspiration/cutting ability of the vitreous instrument; nevertheless, in emergency situations a pars plana paracentesis may be entertained in the office setting. Almost always, however, in such an emergency situation it may be necessary to wait the required preparation time to undertake a more controlled surgical evacuation of vitreous material in the operating room. A more complete core vitrectomy can be achieved in the surgical setting yielding both diagnostic and therapeutic benefit to the patient. This allows more vitreous material to be obtained for better diagnosis, especially where cellular elements are required (i.e., large-cell lymphoma, fungal endophthalmitis).

Cytologic Examination of the Aqueous and Vitreous

Cytologic examination of the aqueous and vitreous obtained on paracentesis may be performed by a number of different methods. The simplest method consists of placing a small drop of fluid from the aspirating needle directly onto the glass slide. Spreading of the drop is not advised since this may disperse the cells too widely. The drop is merely allowed to air dry. When dry, the preparation is fixed in absolute methanol for 10 minutes and once again allowed to dry. The slide is finally placed in dilute buffered Giemsa solution and allowed to stain for 1 hour. It is quickly rinsed with 95% ethanol and allowed to dry. A cover slip is mounted with Canada balsam, and the preparation is examined microscopically. The relative numbers of lymphocytes, polymorphonuclear leukocytes, and macrophages can be determined immediately. In viral infections and chronic hypersensitivity reactions, the cell type is predominantly mononuclear. In acute uveitic reactions, especially those involving the binding of complement to immune complexes (as in Behçet's syndrome), an abundance of neutrophils may be expected, and aqueous and vitreous can be examined by the Raji immune complex assay to determine the amount of immune complex in those fluids. In lens-induced uveitis, one may expect to see many macrophages as well as some neutrophils. In parasitic infections, numerous eosinophils may be seen (see Fig. 2-4). Bacteria or other organisms can be detected by the same examination. If bacteria are seen on the Giemsa preparation, a Gram stain should also routinely be performed on another single drop preparation in the same fashion as has been described (see Figs. 2-8, 2-9, 2-10).

Concentration of Cells and Preparation for Electron Microscopy

Other methods of cytologic examination include techniques for concentrating the cellular elements. The simplest of these consists of passing the entire aspirate through a millipore filter (mean pore size equals 0.45 microns). The filter disk may be stained and cleared with xylene before it is examined microscopically. Various centrifuges have been designed for the concentration of aqueous cells.

Immediately upon aspiration, the cells should be fixed in a glutaraldehyde-paraformaldehyde mixture and postfixed in osmium tetroxide. They are centrifuged onto a thin sheet of araldite before sectioning. This technique results in the preservation of excellent cytologic detail. The secretory granules of the various types of polymorphonuclear leukocytes are easily identifiable and organelles such as the Golgi apparatus can be readily seen. This technique also provides a method for examining viral inclusions in certain cells.

Papanicolaou Technique

The method for the wet fixation of cells by a modification of the Papanicolaou technique may provide an ideal means of identifying intranuclear intracytoplasmic inclusions in affected cells. Studies have indicated that this method is far superior to the Giemsa technique for this purpose.

Identification of *Treponema Pallidum*

Dark field microscopic examinations of aqueous humor specimens have sparked much interest. Smith and co-workers[18] have identified mobile *Treponema* in the aqueous humor of patients suspected of having syphilitic uveitis. Correlative tests, using fluorescent antibody methods, seemed at first to confirm the pathogenic *T. pallidum* in the anterior chamber of these patients but subsequent examinations, with adequately absorbed antisera, seemed to indicate that some of the spirochetal forms observed previously were nonpathogenic treponemas, for example, *Treponema microdentium*. The dark field method is characterized by other difficulties, including the length of time necessary for observation and the frequent appearance of artifacts.

Serologic Examinations of Aqueous and Vitreous Humor

The use of paracentesis for the procurement of diagnostic samples for serologic testing is increasing. Microtiter methods for virtually all the serologic tests used in the laboratory are being perfected for microtiter specimens (Table 2-2). These are available for the testing of aqueous humor and liquid vitreous samples and are particularly useful when tests of the aqueous or vitreous are performed in conjunction with simultaneous tests on the patient's serum.

The ciliary body and iris may act as local factories for the production of antibodies. Whenever it can be established that the specific antibodies detected in the aqueous or vitreous are actually being made in the eye, this has pertinent diagnostic significance. One must also remember that the malignant B cell seen in the eye in large-cell lymphoma (reticulum cell sarcoma) may be identified by the presence of antibodies on its surface (Figs. 2-5, 2-18, 2-19, and 2-20). One can

(*Text continues on p. 43.*)

TABLE 2-2. Intra-ocular Inflammation Serology Measured in Microtiter Quantity

Cytomegalovirus	Ab:CF, IgG and IgM EIA, IgM AbIFA CMV, mRNA, cDNA probe/ISU
Herpes simplex (HSV)	Ab, CF, IgG-EIA IgM-IFA
Histoplasma	Ab, CF, Ag-EIA, Ab-CIE
HTLV-III/LAV	Ab:EIA, IFA, Ag:EIA
Filaria	Ab:CIE, EIA, IFA Ag:Giemsa
Treponema pallidum	VDRL, RPR, FSA-ABS, FTA-ABS-IgM, MHA-TP, Ab-Ay4D, EIA
Sarcoidosis	ACE, V Serum lysozyoid (angiotension converting enzyme)
Leptospira	Ab:CF, IHA, IgG and IgM Ab, EIA
Mumps	Ab:soluble Ag, CF IgM and IgG Ag, viral Ag, CF, IgM and IgG Ab, EIA
Mycobacteria, leprae	Ab and IgM and IgG Ab, EIA
Mycobacteria, Tbc.	Ab: IgG, EIA
Pneumocystis carinii	Ab: IFA, EIA, Ag CIE
Pseudomonas	Ab: CF, IHA, CIE
Strongyloides stercoralis	IgG and IgE Ab, EIA
Subacute Sclerosing Parencephalitis (SSPE)	Measles Antibody Index
Toxocara canis	IgG, IgM, IgA Ab EIA, ELISA
Toxoplasma gondii	IgG, IgM Ab EIA, ELISA Ab: CF, IHA Total and IgM Ab:IFA
Trypanisoma cruzi	Ab: IHA, CF, IFA Total (CSF) IgM:EIA
Varicella Zoster	Ab:CF, IgG and IgM, Ab, EIA
Cryptococcus neoformans	Ag:LPA Ab:IPA
Coccidioides immitis	Ab CF, EIA, ID Ag RIA/EIA

Ab	antibody
ag	antigen
CIE	countercurrent immunoelectrophosis
EIA	enzymal immunoassay
ELISA	enzymal linked immunosorbent assay
CF	complement fraction
IHA	indirect hemagglutination
IFA	indirect fluorescent antibody
ID	immunodiffusion

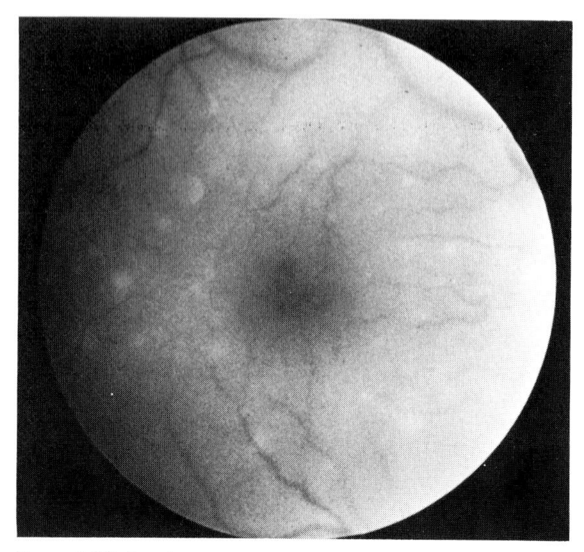

Figure 2-20. Fundus photograph demonstrating blunted retinal details due to overlying vitritis of malignant infiltration of large cell lymphoma. Note white subretinal infiltration of tumor cells in this clinical picture. Vitreous aspiration from this patient yielded a very cellular content to the fluid, making possible a ready diagnosis.

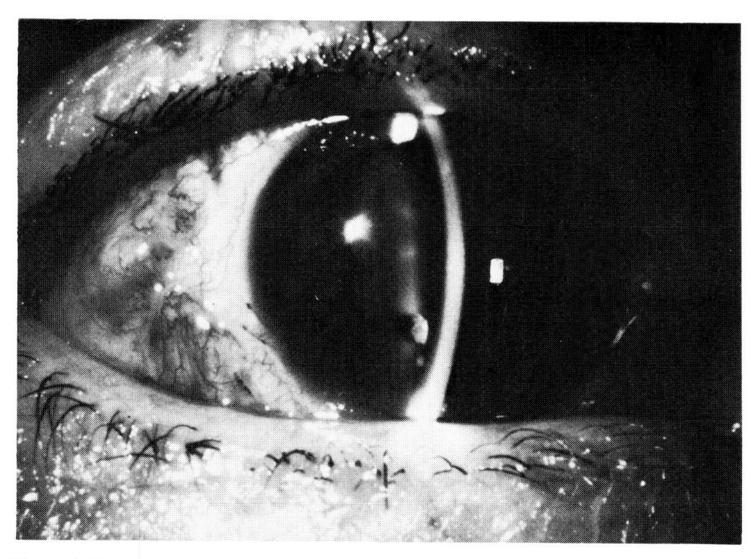

Figure 2-21. Inferior cyclectomy in a patient with atypical ciliary body melanoma, in whom the advanced surgical technique employing a "Peyman" eye basket for stability of the globe allowed for retention of a useful eye.

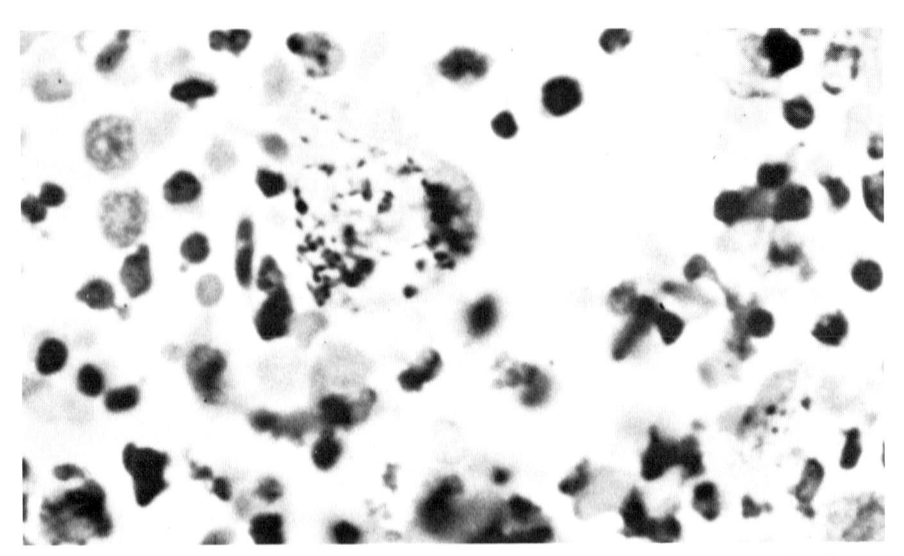

Figure 2-22. Aqueous aspirate of the patient in Figure 2-18 shows an abundance of malignant melanoma cells, which demonstrate the etiology of the masquerade inflammation. This patient had metastatic malignant melanoma from the back to the iris in several foci.

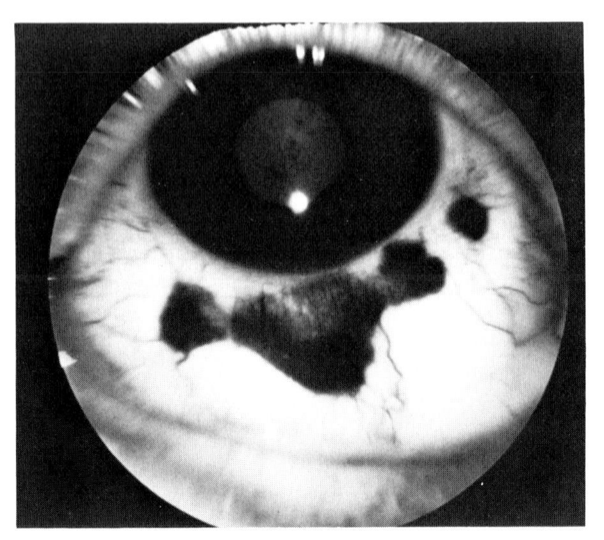

Figure 2-23. Ring melanoma of the ciliary body in a patient with a dense anterior chamber inflammation as noted by background illumination in the anterior chamber.

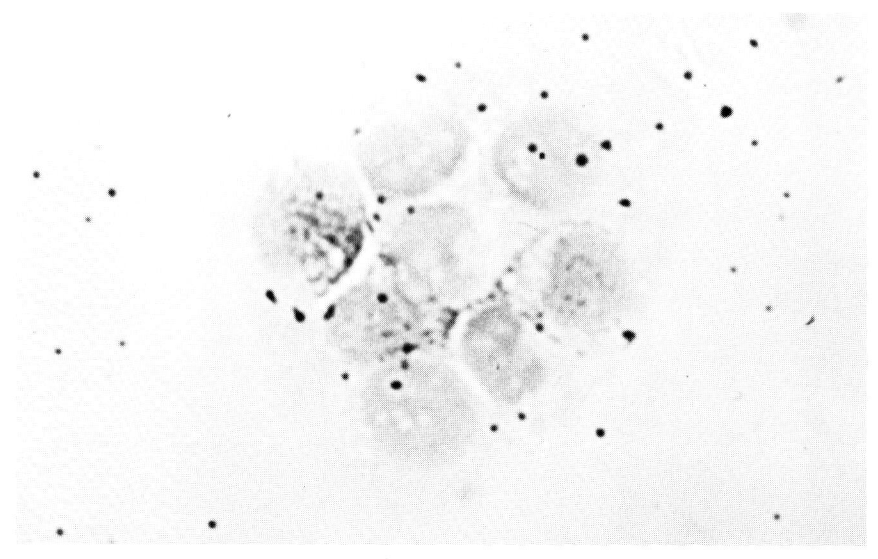

Figure 2-24. Aqueous aspirate of the patient in Figure 2-23 shows a very densely cellular panorama of malignant melanoma cells.

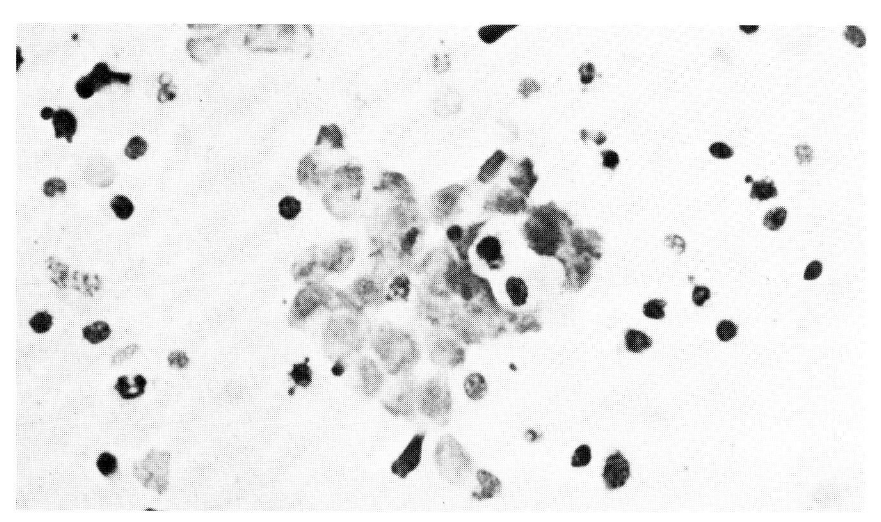

Figure 2-25. Aqueous aspiration from a 2-year-old child thought to have endogenous endophthalmitis reveals retinoblastoma cells amid cellular debris and occasional polymorphonuclear leukocytes.

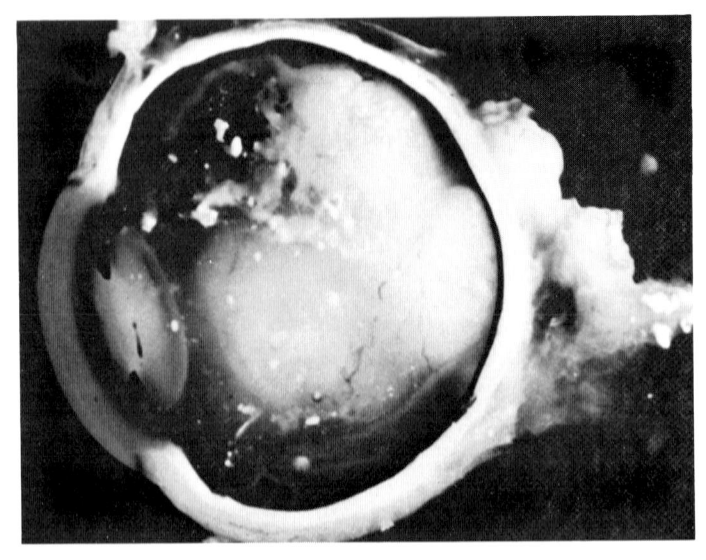

Figure 2-26. Pathologic specimen of eyeball demonstrates the diffuse endophytic retinoblastoma filling almost the entire vitreous cavity with tumor material, some with liquefaction and necrosis, which presented as a clinical diagnostic dilemma until paracentesis of the aqueous revealed the malignant retinoblastoma cells.

demonstrate exclusively Kappa or Lambda light chains that are being produced on these cells as a manifestation of monoclonal infiltration. This is quite different from what would be seen in a mixture of both Kappa and Lambda light chains as manifested in a pure inflammation.

Numerous qualitative reactions are also available for detection of specific antibodies in the aqueous and the vitreous, and these have been adapted to microtiter quantitation by serial dilutions. These include paths of hemoglutination reactions for tuberculosis and, more frequently, ELISA (enzyme linked immunosorbent assay) that have been developed for toxoplasmosis, toxocariasis, and the herpesviruses and are now available for most infectious pathogens. Angiotensin converting enzyme (diagnostic of granulomatous inflammation in general, suggestive of sarcoidosis in particular) can now be measured on such small amounts as aqueous specimens as well.

No chapter on paracentesis of the eye would be complete without mention of "sampling" of the uveal tissue to rule out certain malignancies. While nodules of the iris may be benign in nature, and a consequence of inflammation as well as metaplasia/neoplasia,[19–24] these lesions are more readily accessible for biopsy than choroidal/ciliary body lesions. Pioneering techniques of sophisticated biopsy surgery, initiated by Peyman, have lent themselves to "eye wall biopsy," leaving intact a hitherto candidate for possible enucleation/histopathologic evaluation. These specific surgical techniques have included iridocyclectomy (Fig. 2-21), iridochoroidectomy, eye wall resection, eye wall biopsy, and *ab interno* retinochoroidectomy.[25] These techniques are especially valuable in the difficult diagnoses of large-cell lymphoma infiltrate (see Fig. 2-19), atypical malignant melanoma of the choroid (Figs. 2-22, 2-23, 2-24), therapeutic removal of malignant melanoma of choroid/ciliary body (see Fig. 2-11), atypical retinoblastoma (Figs. 2-25, 2-26), and metastatic cancer of the choroid.

References

1. Bruckner A: Cytologische Studien am Auge. Albrecht von Graefes Arch Klin Opththalmol 100:179, 1919
2. Witmer R: Clinical implications of aqueous humor studies in uveitis. Am J Ophthalmol 86:39, 1978
3. O'Connor GR: Antitoxoplasma precipitins in aqueous humor: New application of the agar diffusion technique. Arch Ophthalmol 57:52, 1957
4. Witmer R: Experimental leptospiral uveitis in rabbits. Arch Ophthalmol 53:547, 1955
5. O'Connor GR: Precipitating antibody to toxoplasma: Follow up study on findings in the blood and aqueous humor. Am J Ophthalmol 44:75, 1957
6. Michelson JB, Belmont JB, Higginbottom P: Juxtapapillary choroiductis associated with chronic meningitis due to coccidioides immitis. Ann Ophthalmol 15:666–668, 1983
7. Allansmith MR, Skaggs C, Kimura SJ: Anterior chamber paracentesis: Diagnostic value in postoperative endophthalmitis. Arch Ophthalmol 84:745, 1970
8. Foster RK: Etiology and diagnosis of bacterial postoperative endophthalmitis. Ophthalmology 85:320–326, 1978
9. Engel H, de la Cruz ZC, Jimenenz-Abalahin LD et al: Cytopreparatory techniques for eye fluid specimens obtained by vitrectomy. Acta Cytol (in press)
10. Brucker AJ, Michels RG, Green WR: Pars plana vitrectomy in the management of blood-induced glaucoma with vitreous hemorrhage. Ann Ophthalmol 10:1427–1437, 1978
11. Brunner WE, Stark WJ, Green WR: Juvenile xanthogranuloma of the iris and ciliary body in an adult. Arch Ophthalmol (submitted for publication)
12. Stark WJ, Rosenthal AR, Mullins GM et al: Simultaneous bilateral uveal melanomas responding to BCNU therapy. Trans Am Acad Ophthalmol Otolaryngol 75:70–83, 1971
13. Piro P, Erozan YS, Michels RG et al: Metastatic breast carcinoma to the vitreous diagnosed by study of pars plana vitrectomy specimen. Ann Ophthalmol (submitted for publication)
14. Michelson JB, Whitaker JP, Wilson S et al: Possible foreign body granuloma of the retina associated with intravenous cocaine addiction. Am J Ophthalmol 887:278–280, 1979
15. Michelson JB, Freedman SD, Boyden DG: Aspergillus endophthalmitis in a drug abuser. Ann Ophthalmol 14:1051–1054, 1982

16. Michelson JB, Roth AM, Waring GO: Lepromatous iridocyclitis diagnosed by anterior chamber paracentesis. Am J Ophthalmol 88:674–679, 1979
17. Michelson JB, Felberg NT, Shields JA et al: Subretinal fluid examination of LDH, PGI, and CEA in a case of metastatic bronchogenic carcinoma of the choroid CA, CCR. 41:2301–2304, 1978
18. Smith JL: The presence of treponemes in aqueous humor in human uveitis. In Aronson SB et al (eds): Clinical Methods in Uveitis, p 159. St Louis, Mosby, 1968
19. Morgan WE III, Malmgren RA, Albert DM: Metastatic carcinoma of the ciliary body simulating uveitis: Diagnosis by cytologic examination of aqueous humor. Arch Ophthalmol 83:54–58, 1970
20. Scholz R, Green WR, Baranano EC et al: Metastatic carcinoma to the iris: Diagnosis by aqueous paracentesis and response to irradiation and chemotherapy. Ophthalmology 90:1524–1527, 1983
21. Takahashi T, Oda Y, Chiba T et al: Metastatic carcinoma of the iris and ciliary body simulating iridocyclitis. Ophthalmologica 188:266–272, 1984
22. Talegaonkar SK: Anterior uveal tract metastasis as the presenting feature of bronchial carcinoma. Br J Ophthalmol 53:123–126, 1969
23. Woog JJ, Chess J, Albert DM et al: Metastatic carcinoma of the iris simulating iridocyclitis. Br J Ophthalmol 68:167–173, 1984
24. Peyman GA, Raichand M, Schulman S: Diagnosis and therapeutic surgery of the uvea. Part I: Surgical technique. Ophthalmol Surg 17:822–829, 1987
25. Denslow GT, Kielar RA: Metastatic adenocarcinoma to the anterior uvea and increased carcinoembryonic antigen levels. Am J Ophthalmol 85:363–367, 1978

Bibliography

Adler B, Faine S: The antibodies involved in the human immune response to leptospiral infection. J Med Microbiol 11:387–400, 1978

Adler B, Murphy AM, Locarnini SA et al: Detection of specific anti-leptospiral immunoglobulins M and G in human serum by solid-phase enzyme-linked immunosorbent assay. J Clin Microbiol 11:452–457, 1980

Affronti LF: Useful immunologic tests for tuberculosis. Clin Immunol Newsletter 4:55–57, 1985

Ambroise-Thomas P: Filariasis. In Houba V (ed): Practical Methods in Clinical Immunology. 2:84–103, 1980

Ambroise-Thomas P: Immunological diagnosis of human filariases: Present possibilities, difficulties and limitations. Acta Tropica 31:108–128, 1974

Ashdown LR: Relationship and significance of specific immunoglobulin M antibody response in clinical and subclinical melioidosis. J Clin Microbiol 14:361–364, 1981

Au-Young JK, Troy FA, Goldstein E: Serologic analysis of antigen-specific reactivity in patients with systemic candidiasis. Diagn Microbiol Infect Dis 3:419–432, 1985

Baker LA, Cox CD: Quantitative assay for genus-specific leptospiral antigena and antibody. Appl Microbiol 25:697–698, 1973

Balestrino EA, Daniel TM, de Latini MDS et al: Serodiagnosis of pulmonary tuberculosis in Argentina by enzyme-linked immunosorbent assay (ELISA) of IgG antibody to

Mycobacterium tuberculosis antigen 5 and tuberculin purified protein derivative. Bull WHO 62:755–761, 1984

Belmont JB, Michelson JB, Bordin GM: Ocular inflammations associated with chronic lymphocytic leukemia. J Ocular Ther and Surg 4:125–129, 1985

Biglan AW, Glickman LT, Lobes LA: Serum and vitreous *Toxocara* antibody in nematode endophthalmitis. Am J Ophthalmol 88:898–901, 1979

Boctor FN, Girgis NS, Elias G et al: A highly sensitive and specific antigen capture EIA for diagnosis of tuberculous meningitis. (in preparation, 1986)

Bowden RA, Sayers M, Flournoy N et al: Cytomegalovirus immune globulin and seronegative blood products to prevent primary cytomegalovirus infection after marrow transplantation. New Engl J Med 314:1006–1010, 1986

Brown ST, Zaidi A, Larsen SA et al: Serological response to syphilis treatment. A new analysis of old data. JAMA 253:1296–1299, 1985

Burnie JP, Williams JD: Evaluation of the Ramco latex agglutination test in the early diagnosis of systemic candidiasis. Eur J Clin Microbiol 4:98–101, 1985

Campbell CK, Payne AL, Teall AJ et al: Cryptococcal latex antigen test positive in patient with Trichosporon beigelii infection. Lancet 2:43–44, 1985

Campbell DG, Essignmann EM: Hemolytic ghost cell glaucoma: further studies. Arch Ophthalmol 97:2141–2146, 1979

Campbell DG, Simmons RJ, Grant WM: Ghost cells as a cause of glaucoma. Am J Ophthalmol 81:441–450, 1976

Cerny EH, Hambie EA, Lee F et al: Adenovirus ELISA for the evaluation of cerebrospinal fluid in patients with suspected neurosyphilis. Am J Clin Path 84:505–508, 1985

Cho S-N, Hunter SW, Gelber RH: Quantitation of the phenolic glycolipid of Mycobacterium leprae and relevance to glycolipid antigen in leprosy. J Infect Dis 153:560–569, 1986

Cho S-N, Yanagihara DL, Hunter SW et al: Serological specificity of phenolic glycolipid I from Mycobacterium leprae and use in serodiagnosis of leprosy. Infect Immun 41:1077–1083, 1983

Clayton AJ, Lisella RS, Martin DG: Melioidosis: A serological survey in military personnel. Milit Med 138:24–26, 1973

Corey L, Spear PG: Infections with herpes simplex viruses. N Engl J Med 314:686–691, 749–757, 1986

Cox RA, Huppert M, Starr P et al: Reactivity of alkali-soluble water-soluble cell wall antigen of C. immitis with anti-coccidioides immunoglobulin M precipitin antibody. Infect Immun 43:502–507, 1984

Cushion MT, Walzer PD: Cultivation of Pneumocystis carinii in lung-derived cell lines. J Infect Dis 149:644, 1984

Cypess RH, Karol MH, Zidian JL et al: Larva-specific antibodies in patients with visceral larva migrans. J Infect Dis 135:633–640, 1977

de Juan E, Rice TA, Green WR et al: Ocular involvement in leukemia. (in preparation)

Demmler GJ, Six HR, Hurst SM et al: Enzyme-linked immunosorbent assay for the detection of IgM-class antibodies to cytomegalovirus. J Infect Dis 153:1152–1155, 1986

Denslow GT, Kielar RA: Metastatic adenocarcinoma to the anterior uvea and increased carcinoembryonic antigen levels. Am J Ophthalmol 85:363–367, 1978

de Repentigny L, Marr LD, Keller JW et al: Comparison of enzyme immunoassay and

gas-liquid chromatography for the rapid diagnosis of invasive candidiasis in cancer patients. J Clin Microbiol 23:46–52, 1986
de Repentigny L, Reiss E: Current trends in immunodiagnosis of candidiasis and aspergillosis. Rev Infect Dis 6:301–312, 1984
de Savigny DH: In vitro maintenance of Toxocara canis larvae and a simple method for production of Toxocara ES antigen for use in serodiagnostic tests for visceral larva migrans. J Parasitol 61:781–782, 1975
Devillechabrolle A, Hugues-Dorin F, Fortier B et al: Prevalence of serum antibodies to herpes simplex virus types 1 and 2: Application of an ELISA technique to 100 cases of anogenital herpes. Sex Trans Dis 12:40–43, 1985
Doft BH, Clarkson JG, Rebell G et al: Endogenous aspergillus endophthalmitis in drug abusers. Arch Ophthalmol 98:859–874m, 1980
Editorial: The lymphatic filariases. Lancet 2:1135–1136, 1985
Editorial: Serological tests for leprosy. Lancet 1:533–535, 1986
Einstein HE: Coccidioidomycosis of central nervous system. Adv Neurol 6:101–105, 1974
Elliot DL, Tolle SW, Goldverg L et al: Pet-associated diseases. N Engl J Med 313:985–995, 1985
Epstein DL, Jedzuniak JA, Grant WM: Identification of heavy-molecular-weight soluble lens protein in aqueous humor in human phacolytic glaucoma. Invest Ophthalmol 17:398–402, 1978
Epstein DL, Jedzuniak JA, Grant WM: Obstruction of aqueous outflow by lens particles and by heavy-molecular-weight soluble lens proteins. Invest Ophthalmol 17:272–277, 1978
Farshy CE, Hunter EF, Helsel LO et al: Four-step enzyme-linked immunosorbent assay for detection of Treponema pallidum antibody. J Clin Microbiol 21:387–389, 1985
Feingold DS, Oski F: Pseudomonas infection: Treatment with immune human plasma. Arch Intern Med 116:326–328, 1965
Ferry AP, Lieberman TW: Bilateral amyloidosis of the vitreous body. Arch Ophthalmol 94:982–991, 1976
Flocks M, Littwin CS, Zimmerman LE: Phacolytic glaucoma. Arch Ophthalmol 54:37–45, 1955
Forghani B, Schmidt NJ, Dennis J: Antibody assays for varicella-zoster virus: Comparison of enzyme immunoassay with neutralization, immune adherence hemagglutination, and complement fixation. J Clin Microbiol 8:545–552, 1978
Freeman R, Hamblin MH: Serological studies on 40 cases of mumps virus infection. J Clin Pathol 33:28–32, 1980
Fujita S, Matsubara F, Matsuda T: Enzyme-linked immunosorbent assay measurement of fluctuations in antibody titer and antigenemia in cancer patients with and without candidiasis. J Clin Microbiol 23:568–575, 1986
Galgiani JN, Dugger KO, Ito JI et al: Antigenemia in primary coccidioidomycosis. Am J Trop Med Hyg 33:645–649, 1984
Gallo D, Diggs JL, Shell GR et al: Comparison of detection of antibody to the acquired immune deficiency syndrome virus by enzyme immunoassay, immunofluorescence, and western blot methods. J Clin Microbiol 23:1049–1051, 1986
Gershon AA, Steinberg SP, Gelb L et al: Clinical reinfection with varicell-zoster virus. J Infect Dis 149:137–142, 1984
Glickman LT, Grieve RB, Lauria SS et al: Serodiagnosis of ocular toxocariasis: A comparison of two antigens. J Clin Pathol 38:103–107, 1985

Glickman LT, Grieve RB, Schantz PM: Serologic diagnosis of zoonotic pulmonary dirofilariasis. Am J Med 80:161–164, 1986
Glickman LT, Schantz P, Dombroske R et al: Evaluation of serodiagnostic tests for visceral larva migrans. Am J Trop Med Hyg 67:24–28, 1979
Goldberg MF: Cytological diagnosis of phacolytic glaucoma utilizing millipore filtration of the aqueous. Br J Ophthalmol 51:847–853, 1967
Goodman JS, Kaufman L, Koenig MG: Diagnosis of cryptococcal meningitis: Value of immunologic detection of cryptococcal antigen. N Engl J Med 285:434–436, 1971
Goudsmit J, deWolf F, Paul DA et al: Expression of human immunodifficiency virus antigen (HIV-Ag) in serum and cerebrospinal fluid during acute and chronic infection. Lancet 2:177–180, 1986
Green WR, Kenyon KR, Michels RG et al: Ultrastructure of epiretinal membranes causing macular pucker after retinal reattachment surgery. Trans Ophthalmol Soc UK 99:63–77, 1979
Gut J-P, Spiess C, Schmitt S et al: Rapid diagnosis of acute mumps infection by a direct immunoglobulin M antibody capture enzyme immunoassay with labeled antigen. J Clin Microbiol 21:346–352, 1985
Hall SM: The diagnosis of toxoplasmosis. Brit Med J 289:570–571, 1984
Hamilton RG: Application of immunoassay methods in the serodiagnosis of human filariasis. Rev Infect Dis 7:837–843, 1985
Izzat NN, Bartruff JK, Glicksman JM et al: Validity of the VDRL test on cerebrospinal fluid contaminated by blood. Brit J Vener Dis 47:162–164, 1971
Joassin L, Reginster M: Elimination of nonspecific cytomegalovirus immunoglobulin M activities in the enzyme-linked immunosorbent assay by using anti-human immunoglobulin G. J Clin Microbiol 23:576–581, 1986
Johnson RT, Olson LC, Buescher EL: Herpes simplex virus infections of the nervous system: Problems in laboratory diagnosis. Arch Neurol 18:260–264, 1968
Jones CE, Alexander JW, Fisher M: Clinical evaluation of Pseudomonas hyperimmune globulin. J Surg Res 14:87–96, 1973
Jones RJ, Roe EA, Gupta JL: Controlled trials of a polyvalent Pseudomonas vaccine in burns. Lancet 2:977–983, 1979
Jones RJ, Roe EA, Lowbury EJL et al: A new Pseudomonas vaccine: Preliminary trial on human volunterers. J Hyg (Camb) 76:429–439, 1976
Kadival GV, Mazarelo TBMS, Chapras SD: Sensitivity and specificity of enzyme-linked immunosorbent assay in the detection of antigen in tuberculous meningitis cerebrospinal fluids. J Clin Microbiol 23:901–904, 1986
Kagan IG: Diagnostic, epidemiologic, and experimental parasitology: Immunologic aspects. Am J Trop Med Hyg 28:429–439, 1979
Kahn FW, Jones JM: Latex agglutination tests for detection of candida antigens in sera of patients with invasive candidiasis. J Infect Dis 153:579–585, 1986
Kampik A, Green WR, Michels RG: Ultrastructural features of progressive idiopathic epiretinal membrane removed by vitreous surgery. Am J Ophthalmol 90:797–809, 1980
Karam GH, Griffitn FM Jr: Invasive pulmonary aspergillosis in nonimmunocomprised, nonneutropenic hosts. Rev Infect Dis 8:357–363, 1986
Kaufman L, Standard PG, Huppert M et al: Comparison and diagnostic value of the coccidioidin heat-stable (HS and tube precipitin) antigens in immunodiffusion. J Clin Microbiol 22:515–518, 1985

Kaushal NA, Hussain R, Ottesen EA: Excretory-secretory and somatic antigens in the diagnosis of human filariasis. Clin Exp Immunol 56:567–576, 1984
Kenyon DR, Pederson JE, Green WR et al: Fibroglial proliferation in pars planitis. Trans Ophthalmol Soc UK 95:391–397, 1975
Kinney JS, Onorato IM, Stewart JA et al: Cytomegaloviral infection and disease. J Infect Dis 151:772–774, 1985
Klingele TG, Hogan MJ: Ocular reticulum cell sarcoma. Am J Ophthalmol 79:39–47, 1975
Kovacs JA, Gill V, Swan JC et al: Prospective evaluation of a monoclonal antibody in diagnosis of Pneumocystis carinii pneumonia. Lancet 2:1–3, 1986
Krambovitis E, Harris M, Hughes DTD: Improved serodiagnosis of tuberculosis using two assay test. J Clin Path 39:779–785, 1986
Krambovitis E, McIllmurray MB, Lock PE et al: Rapid diagnosis of tuberculous meningitis by latex particle agglutination. Lancet 2:1229–1231, 1984
Larson SA, Hambie EA, Wobig GH et al: Cerebrospinal fluid serologies in syphilis: Treponemal and nontreponemal tests. International Conjoint S.T.D. meeting, Montreal, Canada. Abstract 166:218, 1984
Lee FK, Nahmias AJ, Stagno S: Rapid diagnosis of cytomegalovirus infection in infants by electron microscopy. New Engl J Med 299:1266–1270, 1978
Libertin CR, Woloschak GE, Wilson WR et al: Analysis of Pneumocystis carinii cysts with a fluorescence-activated cell sorter. J Clin Microbiol 20:877–880, 1984
Luft BJ, Conley F, Remington JS et al: Outbreak of central-nervous-system toxoplasmosis in Western Europe and North America. Lancet 1:781–784, 1983
Maddison SE, Walls KW, Haverkos HW et al: Evaluation of serologic tests for Pneumocystis carinii antibody and antigenemia in patients with acquired immunodeficiency syndrome. Diagn Microbiol Infect Dis 2:69–73, 1984
Manning-Zweerink M, Malonmey CS, Mitchell TG et al: Immunoblot analyses of Candida albicans-associated antigens and antibodies in human sera. J Clin Microbiol 23:46–52, 1986
Manschot WA: Persistent hyperplastic primary vitreous. Arch Ophthalmol 59:188–203, 1958
Mardh P-A, Larsson L, Hoiby N et al: Tuberculostearic acid as a diagnostic marker in tuberculous meningitis. Lancet 1:367, 1983
Martin WJ II, Smith TF: Rapid detection of cytomegalovirus in bronchoalveolar lavage specimens by a monoclonal antibody method. J Clin Microbiol 23:1006–1008, 1986
Martinez-Martin P, Garcia-Saiz A, Rapun JL et al: Intrathecal synthesis of IgG antibodies to varicella-zoster virus in two cases of acute aseptic meningitis syndrome with no cutaneous lesions. J Med Virol 16:201–209, 1985
Matthews RC, Burnie JP, Tabaqchali S: Immunoblot analysis of the serological response in systemic candidosis. Lancet 2:1415–1418, 1984
Mayer KH, Stoddard AM, McCusker J et al: Human T-lymphotropic virus type III in high-risk, antibody-negative homosexual men. Ann Intern Med 104:194–196, 1986
McCabe RE, Remington JS: The diagnosis and treatment of toxoplasmosis. Eur J Clin Microbiol 2:95–104, 1983
McHugh TM, Casavant CH, Wilber JC et al: Comparison of six methods for the detection antibody to cytomegalovirus. J Clin Microbiol 22:1014–1019, 1985
McKeating JA, Stagno S, Stirk PR et al: Detection of Cytomegalovirus in urine samples by enzyme-linked immunosorbent assay. J Med Virol 16:367–373, 1985
Melioli G, Pedulla D, Merli AL et al: A simple method to detect intrathecal production of

specific antimeasles antibodies in cerebrospinal fluid during subacute sclerosing panencephalitis. Diagn Microbiol Infect Dis 3:411–417, 1985
Michels RG, Knox DL, Drozan YS et al: Intraocular reticulum cell sarcoma. Arch Ophthalmol 93:1331–1335, 1975
Michelson JB, Chisari FV, Kansu J: Antibodies to oral mucosa in patients with ocular Behçet's disease. Ophthalmol 92:1277–1281, 1985
Michelson JB, Grossman KR, Lozier JR: Iridocyclitis masquerade syndrome. Surg Ophthalmol 31:125–130, 1986
Michelson JB, Michelson PE, Bordin GM et al: Ocular reticulum cell sarcoma presenting as retinal detachment with demonstration of monoclonal immunoglobulin light chains on the vitreous cells. Arch Ophthalmol 99:1409–1411, 1981
Milner AR, Jackson KB, Woodruff K et al: Enzyme-linked immunosorbent assay for determining specific immunoglobulin M in infections caused by Leptospira interrogans serovar hardjo. J Clin Microbiol 22:539–542, 1985
Morgan WE, Malmgren RA, Albert DM: Metastatic carcinoma of the ciliary body simulating uveitis: Diagnosis by cytologic examination of aqueous humor. Arch Ophthalmol 83:54–58, 1970
Morris GE, Coleman RM, Best JM et al: Persistence of serum IgA antibodies to herpes simplex, varicella-zoster, cytomegalovirus, and rubella virus detected by enzyme-lined immunosorbent assays. J Med Biol 16:343–349, 1985
Muller F: Specific immunoglobulin M and G antibodies in the rapid diagnosis of human treponemal infections. Diag Immuno 4:1–9, 1986
Muller F, Moskophidis M: Estimation of the local production of antibodies to Preponema pallidum in the central nervous system of patients with neurosyphilis. Br J Vener Dis 59:80–84, 1983
Nahmias AJ, Whitley RJ, Visintine AN et al: Herpes simplex virus encephalitis: Laboratory evaluations and their diagnostic significance. J Infect Dis 145:829–836, 1982
Nashed H, Peter JB: Melioidosis: Comparison of EIA and IGFA methods for diagnosis. (in preparation, 1986)
Nigro G, Nanni F, Midulla M: Determination of vaccine-induced and naturally acquired class-specific mumps antibodies by two indirect enzyme-linked immunosorbent assays. J Virol Methods 13:91–106, 1986
Novey HS, Wells ID: Allergic bronchopulmonary aspergillosis. West J Med 130:1–5, 1979
Nutman TB, Miller KD, Mulligan M et al: Loa loa infection in temporary residents of endemic regions: Recognition of a hyper-responsive syndrome with characteristic clinical manifestations. J Infect Dis 154:10–17, 1986
O'Donnell FE Jr: Nikon's resident diagnosis of the month. Ophthalmology Times, February 1978
Ottesen EA: Immunological aspects of lymphatic filariasis and onchocerciasis in man. Trans Royal Soc Trop Med Hyg 78(Suppl):9–18, 1984
Panjwani DD, Ball MG, Berry NJ et al: Virological and serological diagnosis of cytomegalovirus infection in bone marrow allograft recipients. J Med Virol 16:357–365, 1985
Pappagianis D: Serology and serodiagnosis of coccidioidomycosis. In Stevens DA (ed): Coccidioidomycosis, pp 97–112. New York, Plenum Publishing, 1980
Parver LM, Font RL: Malignant lymphoma of the retina and brain: Initial diagnosis by cytologic examination of vitreous aspirate. Arch Ophthalmol 97:1505–1507, 1979
Paryani SG, Arvin AM: Intrauterine infection with varicella-zoster virus after maternal varicella. N Engl J Med 314:1542–1546, 1986

Pederson JE, Kenyon KR, Green WR et al: Pathology of pars planitis. Am J Ophthalmol 86:762–774, 1978
Perfect JR, Durack DT, Gallis HA: Cryptococcemia. Medicine 62:98–109, 1983
Peter JB, Devi SJN: Intrathecal synthesis of Coccidioides-specific IgG in coccidioidal meningitis. (unpublished data)
Pettit TH, Olson RJ, Foos RY et al: Fungal endophthalmitis following introcular lens implantation. Arch Ophthalmol 98:1025–1039, 1980
Pitt TLL, Todd HC, Mackintosh CA et al: Evaluation of three serological tests for detection of antibody to Pseudomonas aeruginosa in human sera. Eur J Clin Microbiol 4:190–196, 1985
Price FW, Schlaegel TF: Bilateral acute retinal necrosis. Am J Ophthalmol 89:419–424, 1980
Radolf JD, Lernhardt EB, Fehniger TE et al: Serodiagnosis of syphilis by enzyme-linked immunosorbent assay with purified recombinant Treponema pallidum antigen 4D. J Infect Dis 153:1023–1027, 1986
Redfield RR, Wright DC, Tramont EC: The Walter Reed staging classification for HTLV-III/LAV infection. N Engl J Med 314:131–132, 1986
Reese AB: Persistent hyperplastic primary vitreous. Am J Ophthalmol 40:317–331, 1955
Reeves WC, Corey L, Adams HG et al: Risk of recurrence after first episodes of genital herpes. N Engl J Med 305:315–319, 1981
Reiss E, Cherniak RE, Eby R et al: Enzyme immunoassay detection of IgM to galactoxylomannan of Cryptococcus neoformans. Diag Immunol 2:109–115, 1984
Remky H: Tumorzellen im Kammerwasser. Klin Monatsbl Augenheilkd 138:643–649, 1961
Robertson DM: Metastatic malignant melanoma to vitreous diagnosed by cytologic examination. Personal communication May 19, 1980
Rodman HI, Johnson FB, Zimmerman LE: New histopathological and histochemical observations concerning asteroid hyalitis. Arch Ophthalmol 66:552–563, 1961
Ryan SJ, Maumenee AE: Birdshot retinochoroidopathy. Am J Ophthalmol 89:31–45, 1980
Sabetta JR, Miniter P, Andriole VT: The diagnosis of invasive aspergillosis by an enzyme-linked immunosorbent assay for circulating antigen. J Infect Dis 152:946–953, 1985
Salahuddin SZ, Groopman JE, Markham PD et al: HTLV-III in symptom-free seronegative persons. Lancet 2:1418–1420, 1984
Sandford GR, Merz WG, Wingard JR et al: The value of fungal surveillance cultures as predictors of systemic fungal infections. J Infect Dis 142:503–509, 1980
Schmidt NJ: Further evidence for common antigens in herpes simplex and varicella-zoster virus. J Med Virol 9:27–36, 1982
Schofield PB: Diffuse infiltrating retinoblastoma. Br J Ophthalmol 44:35–41, 1960
Schonheyder H, Andersen P: IgG antibodies to purified Aspergillus fumigatus antigens determined by enzyme-linked immunosorbent assay. Int Archs Allergy Appl Immunol 74:262–269, 1984
Schrier RD, Nelson JA, Oldstone MBA: Detection of human cytomegalovirus in peripheral blood lymphocytes in a natural infection. Science 230:1048–1051, 1985
Schuster V, Matz B, Wiegand H et al: Detection of human cytomegalovirus in urine by DNA-DNA and RNA-DNA hybridization. J Infect Dis 154:309–314, 1986
Schwartz MF, Green WR, Michels RG: Case report. Ophthalmology (submitted for publication)

Sever JL, Jacob AJ: Laboratory diagnosis of herpesvirus infections. Seminars in Perinatology 7:57–63, 1983
Shanley J, Myers M, Edmond B et al: Enzyme-linked immunosorbent assay for detection of antibody to varicella-zoster virus. J Clin Microbiol 15:208–211, 1982
Shields JA, Lerner HA, Felberg NT: Aqueous cytology and enzymes in nematode endophthalmitis. Am J Ophthalmol 84:319–322, 1977
Shuster EA, Beneke JS, Tegtmeier GE et al: Monoclonal antibody for rapid laboratory detection of cytomegalovirus infections: Characterization and diagnostic application. Mayo Clin Proc 60:577–585, 1985
Snip RC, Michels RG: Pars plana vitrectomy in the management of endogenous Candida endophthalmitis. Am J Ophthalmol 82:699–704, 1976
Speiser F: Application of the enzyme-linked immunosorbent assay (ELISA) for the diagnosis of filariasis and echinococcosis. Tropenmed Parasit 31:459–466, 1980
Stagno S, Tinker MK, Elrod C et al: Immunoglobulin M antibodies detected by enzyme-linked immunosorbent assay and radioimmunoassay in the diagnosis of cytomegalovirus infections in pregnant women and newborn infants. J Clin Microbiol 21:930–935, 1985
Stagno S, Whitley RJ: Herpes virus infections of pregnancy. Part I: Cytomegalovirus and Epstein-Barr virus infections. New Engl J Med 313:1270–1274, 1985
Stark WJ, Michels RG, Maumenee AE et al: Surgical management of epithelial ingrowth. Am J Ophthalmol 85:772–780, 1980
Stockman L, Roberts GD: Corrected version: Specificity of the latex test for cryptococcal antigen: A rapid, simple method for eliminating interference factors. J Clin Microbiol 17:945–947, 1983
Straus E, Wu N, Quraishi MAH et al: Clinical applications of the radioimmunoassay of secretory tuberculoprotein. Proc Natl Acad Sci USA 78:3214–3217, 1981
Straus SE, Rooney JF, Sever JL et al: Herpes simplex virus infection: Biology, treatment, and prevention. Ann Intern Med 103:404–419, 1985
Sulzer CR, Jones WL: Evaluation of a hemagglutination test for human leptospirosis. Appl Microbiol 26:655–657, 1973
Tanabe K, Furuta T, Ueda K et al: Serological observations of Pneumocystis carinii infection in humans. J Clin Microbiol 22:1058–1060, 1985
Taylor HR: Report of a workshop: Research priorities for immunologic aspects of onchocerciasis. J Infect Dis 152:389–394, 1985
Terpstra WJ, Ligthart GS, Schoone GJ: Sero diagnosis of human leptospirosis by enzyme-linked-immunosorbent assay (ELISA). Zbl Bakt Hyg, I. Abt Orig A 247:400–405, 1980
Theodore FH: Etiology and diagnosis of fungal postoperative endophthalmitis. Ophthalmology 85:327–339, 1978
Trachtman H, Hammerschlag MR, Tejani A et al: A longitudinal study of varicella immunity in pediatric renal transplant recipients. J Infect Dis 154:335–337, 1985
Trull AK, Parker J, Warren RE: IgG enzyme linked immunosorbent assay for diagnosis of invasive aspergillosis: retrospective study over 15 years of transplant recipients. J Clin Pathol 38:1045–1051, 1985
Turner LH: Leptospirosis II: Serology. Trans Roy Soc Trop Med Hyg 62:880–899, 1968
Ukkonen P, Granstrom M-L, Penttinen K: Mumps-specific immunoglobulin M and G antibodies in natural mumps infection as measured by enzyme-linked immunosorbent assay. J Med Virol 8:131–142, 1981

Ukkonen P, Granstrom M-L, Rasanen J et al: Local production of mumps IgG and IgM antibodies in the cerebrospinal fluid of meningitis patients. J Med Virol 8:257–265, 1981

Vandvik B, Nilsen RE, Vartdal F et al: Mumps meningitis: Specific and non-specific antibody responses in the central nervous system. Acta Neurol Scand 65:468–487, 1982

van Knapen F, Panggabean SO, van Leusden J: Demonstration of Toxoplasma antigen containing complexes in active toxoplasmosis. J Clin Microbiol 22:645–650, 1985

Verhoeff FH: Microscopic findings in a case of asteroid hyalitis. Am J Ophthalmol 4:155–160, 1921

Wagoner MD, Goner JR, Albert DM et al: Intraocular reticulum cell sarcoma. Ophthalmology 87:724–727, 1980

Waitkins S: Laboratory diagnosis of leptospirosis. Laboratory Technology 17:178–184, 1983

Walls KW, Wilson M: Immunoserology in parasitic infections. In Aloisi RM, Hyun J (eds): Immunodiagnostics, pp 191–214. New York, Alan R, Liss, 1983

Weiner MH: Antigenemia detected in human coccidioidomycosis. J Clin Microbiol 18:136–142, 1983

Weiner MH, Talbot GH, Gerson SL et al: Antigen detection in the diagnosis of invasive aspergillosis. Utility in controlled, blinded trials. Ann Intern Med 99:777–7821, 1983

Weiss SH, Goedert JJ, Sarngadharan MG et al: Screening test for HTLV-III (AIDS agent) antibodies: Specificity, sensitivity, and applications. JAMA 253:221–225, 1985

Welch PC, Masur H, Jonees TC et al: Serologic diagnosis of acute lymphadenopathic toxoplasmosis. J Infect Dis 142:256–264, 1980

Wheat J, French MLV, Kamel S et al: Evaluation of cross-reactions in Histoplasma capsulatum serologic tests. J Clin Microbiol 23:493–499, 1986

Wheat J, French MLV, Kohler RB et al: The diagnostic laboratory tests for histoplasmosis: Analysis of experience in a large urban outbreak. Ann Intern Med 97:680–685, 1982

Wheat LJ, Kohler RB, Tewari RP: Diagnosis of disseminated histoplasmosis by detection of Histoplasma capsulatum antigen in serum and urine specimens. N Engl J Med 314:83–88, 1986

Whitley RJ, Nahmias AJ, Visintine AM et al: The natural history of herpes simplex virus infection of mother and newborn. Pediatrics 66:489–494, 1980

Wieden MA, Galgiani JN, Pappagianis D: Comparison of immunodiffusion techniques with standard complement fixation assay for quantitation of coccidioidal antibodies. J Clin Microbiol 18:529–534, 1983

Wilkinson CP: Metastatic malignant melanoma to the vitreous and diagnosed by cytologic examination. Personal communication, Dec. 4, 1979. Case also presented by Dr. L.E. Zimmerman at the Verhoeff Society, April 24, 1980

Willerson D, Aaberg TM, Reeser Fh: Necrotizing vaso-occulsive retinitis. Am J Ophthalmol 84:209–219, 1977

Wong-Staal F, Gallo RC: Human T-lymphotrophic retroviruses. Nature 317:395–403, 1985

Wood DJ, Corbitt G: Viral infections in childhood leukemia. J Infect Dis 152:266–273, 1985

Yanez MA, Coppola MP, Russo DA et al: Determination of mycobacterial antigens in sputum by enzyme immunoassay. J Clin Microbiol 23:822–825, 1986

Yanoff M, Scheie HG: Cytology of human lens aspirate. Arch Ophthalmol 80:166–170, 1968

Young NJ, Bird AC: Bilateral acute retinal necrosis. Br J Ophthalmol 62:581–590, 1978

Young DB, Buchanan TM: A serological test for leprosy with a glycolipid specific for Mycobacterium leprae. Science 221:1057–1059, 1983

Young DB, Dissanayake S, Miller RA et al: Humans respond predominantly with IgM immunoglobulin to the species-specific glycolipid of Mycobacterium leprae. J Infect Dis 149:870–873, 1984

Ziegler EJ, McCutchan JA, Fierer J et al: Treatment of gram-negative bacteremia and shock with human antiserum to a mutant Escherichia coli. N Engl J Med 307:1225–1230, 1982

Ziola B, Halonen P, Enders G: Synthesis of measles virus-specific IgM antibodies and IgM-class rheumatoid factor in relation to clinical onset of subacute sclerosing panencephalitis. J Med Virol 18:51–59, 1986

Zuger A, Louie E, Holzman RS et al: Cryptococcal disease in patients with the acquired immunodeficiency syndrome. Ann Intern Med 104:234–240, 1986

THREE

The Immunology of Uveitis

Despite a vast array of etiologies, most observers agree that immune mechanisms play a major role in uveitis. This appears to be the case whether we are dealing with infectious etiologies, such as toxoplasmosis and tuberculosis, or systemic immunologic diseases such as sarcoid, Reiter's syndrome, and ankylosing spondylitis.

We have made substantial progress in understanding why the uveal tract is an active participant in immunologic types of inflammation. But it remains puzzling why it is so often singled out as the main ocular target in widespread, multisystem inflammatory disease. We know, for example, that the uveal tract is one of the most vascular tissues in the entire body, and certainly these vascular channels must provide temporary residence for large numbers of cellular and humoral elements of inflammation. These products may have a nonspecific inflammatory effect, or they may be specifically directed against antigens in the uveal tract.

The participation of the uvea in systemic inflammation has long been recognized by ophthalmologists and immunologists alike. When rats are injected with complete Freund's adjuvant, they develop arthritis and uveal inflammation.[1] Similarly, intraperitoneal injection of protein antigen leads to widespread inflammation of the skin, uvea, and several internal organs.[2]

Histologically, one cannot help but be impressed by the large numbers of mast cells that populate the uveal tract (Fig. 3-1). It is worth noting that the uvea

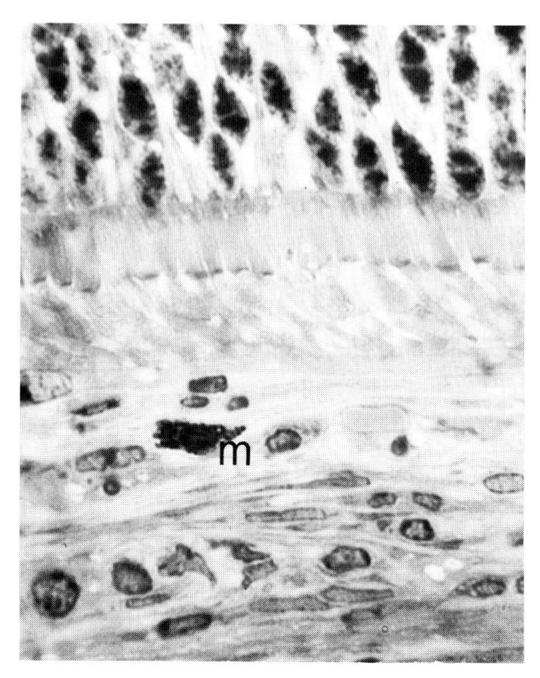

Figure 3-1. Mast cell (*m*) in the uveal tract of a normal guinea pig (Giemsa, original magnification ×1100).

may have a higher concentration of these immunologically important cells than any other tissue.[3,4]

We have suggested that mast cells could regulate the tone of blood vessels and perhaps control the passage of cells in various tissues.[5] Mast cells are very prominent in vascular tissues, and they are intimately associated with blood vessels at the corneal limbus and throughout the uveal tract.

Mast cells are known to contain high concentrations of vasoactive substances such as histamine,[6] and they are active participants in allergic reactions mediated by immunoglobulin E. Mast cells are, in fact, the site for attachment of IgE molecules and there may be tens of thousands of IgE molecules on the surface of a single mast cell. In the typical allergic reaction, a highly specific interaction between antigen and antibody takes place on the surface of a mast cell (Fig. 3-2). This triggers a series of events within the mast cell leading to the release of granular substances such as histamine. A series of parallel events takes place in the mast cell membrane in which other important mediators of inflammation are generated. These substances include prostaglandins, thromboxanes, and leukotrienes. The role of these substances in ocular inflammation is still under investigation.[7] However, it is known that leukotrienes C4 and D4 are 4000 times as potent as histamine in their ability to constrict smooth muscle and dilate blood vessels, and leukotriene B4 is the most potent chemotactic substance known to man.[6]

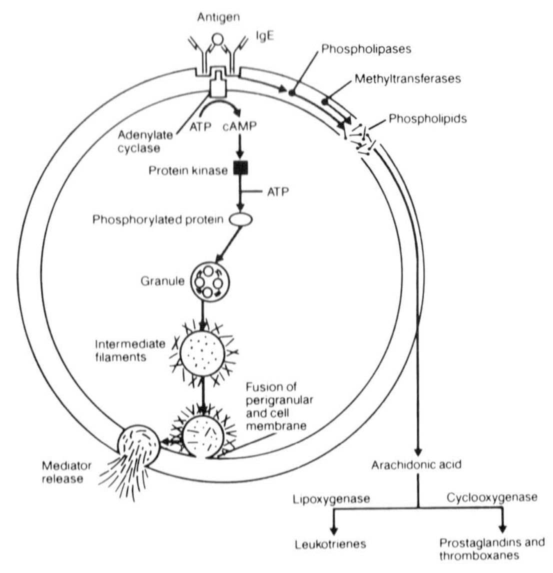

Figure 3-2. Diagram of interaction between antigen and cell-bound IgE, which leads to the release of mast cell granules and generation of arachidonic acid (precursor of prostaglandins, thromboxanes, and leukotrienes). ATP, adenosine triphosphate; cAMP, cyclic adenosine monophosphate. (Adapted, with permission, from Austen[6], p 230; original artist, Bunji Tagawa)

Aside from the presence of fixed tissue cells, large numbers of eosinophils are attracted to the uveal tract, especially after immunologic challenge.[4] Eosinophils have been observed for decades and have long been considered the signature of the allergic reaction. But the function of the eosinophil and its role in ocular disease is poorly understood. Eosinophils are known to contain major basic protein toxic to helminths and to mammalian cells such as respiratory epithelium.[8]

Circumstantial evidence implicates the mast cell and eosinophil as important players in uveal immune responses. Exactly how these cells are triggered and how they interact with antigen or uveal tissue will provide fertile territory for future decades of basic research.

Infectious Causes of Uveitis

Toxoplasmosis

Most infectious types of uveitis result not from direct ocular inoculation but rather from the migration of microorganisms from some distant site in the body.

This is the case with toxoplasmosis where the parasite spreads through the bloodstream and lodges preferentially in the brain and choroid. Most toxoplasma infections are congenital and transmitted to the fetus *in utero* during the first trimester of pregnancy.[9] The parasite produces only a mild flu-like illness in the mother, while the effect on the fetus, whose immune system is immature, may be disastrous. If fetal death and spontaneous abortion do not occur, the infant may be mentally retarded or it may face a lifetime of recurrent uveitis.

This then is a situation in which a ubiquitous organism infects a host with normal immunity and produces a self-limited infection. In an immature immune system, the same organism can cause a much different and more severe disease.

Serologic surveys have demonstrated that up to 50% of the population in the United States has been infected with toxoplasma. Most of these infections are subclinical and often the disease goes unrecognized. Most of the ocular disease associated with toxoplasmosis probably occurs because of reactivation of congenital infections. Factors that compromise the host's ocular immunity may reactivate the dormant infection and lead to a disseminated infection.

Toxoplasma infection stimulates formation of IgG and IgM antibodies, detectable by various serologic techniques. Antibody alone is not sufficient to protect the host from infection. Even in the presence of high levels of antibody, the parasite can persist. Yet the ability of the macrophage to destroy infective trophozoites is greatly enhanced if the toxoplasma organisms are first exposed to antibody and complement or lymphokines. These humoral factors seem to prepare the organisms for phagocytosis by macrophages.

Because of the importance of the lymphocyte-macrophage immune cell axis, drugs that suppress immunity, such as corticosteroids and cytotoxic agents, can induce reactivation of toxoplasmosis causing dissemination of the parasite. For this reason, corticosteroids must be used with extreme caution in toxoplasmosis and in other types of infectious uveitis.

Toxocariasis

Similar mechanisms may play a role in toxocara infection and its systemic counterpart, visceral larva migrans. In this condition, infants who ingest soil contaminated with toxocara organisms can develop widespread foci of parasitic inflammation.[10] The eye, liver, and spleen are preferentially involved. No doubt, a tremendous number of parasitic organisms overwhelm the child's immature immune system and lead to foci of parasitic inflammation, fever, and eosinophilia.

Syphilis

Although syphilitic uveitis is rare today, it is crucial to rule out this diagnosis in evaluating patients with uveitis. This can be done with serologic tests such as the VDRL and FTA-Abs. The former test measures antibodies directed against the spirochete, which cross-reacts with a tissue-derived substance known as *cardioli-*

pin, a component of mitochondrial membranes. The VDRL may become negative when the luetic infection is quiescent, however the FTA-Abs, a fluorescent treponemal antibody test remains positive throughout life.

Many of the pathologic findings in syphilis are the direct result of an exuberant immune responses. Immune complexes may be deposited in the kidneys or other vascular tissues.[11] Immunity to the spirochete depends on a complex of interactions between humoral and cellular factors.

Several lines of evidence suggest the importance of antibody in this infection. But antibodies that develop during the course of syphilitic infection are at best only partially protective. Syphilis progresses through the primary and secondary stages in spite of the presence of antibodies that immobilize treponemes. Cellular immunity is felt to be important in the body's control of this organism. Delayed hypersensitivity directed against treponemal antigens develops late in secondary syphilis but may be absent in primary and early secondary disease.

Tuberculosis

In tuberculosis, cellular immunity is decisive in recovery from infection. The tuberculin skin test, a manifestation of cellular immunity, is useful in making a diagnosis. False-negative tests may occur in disseminated tuberculosis, measles, sarcoidosis, lymphoma, and other conditions that depress cellular immunity. A false-negative test may also be encountered in patients taking corticosteroids or other immunosuppressive drugs.

The organism itself has the ability to survive and proliferate within phagocytic cells. It may evade the usual bactericidal activity of macrophages by preventing the fusion of enzyme-containing lysozymes with phagosomes containing the organisms. The most important form of ocular tuberculosis is that which affects the uveal tract. Either direct infection of the tissues or diffuse hypersensitivity states in previously affected individuals may be seen.

Leprosy

Leprosy, another mycobacterial infection, has many interesting immunologic features. Patients with lepromatous leprosy have impaired cellular immunity against *Mycobacterium leprae.* They demonstrate anergy to the lepromin skin test while normal persons often have a positive delayed hypersensitivity reaction.[12]

Patients with lepromatous leprosy have lower than normal levels of circulating T- and B-lymphocytes and marked depletion of T cells from their lymph nodes. The development of infection is apparently related to the survival of the bacillus within macrophages.

In contrast to the deficits in cellular immunity, patients with lepromatous leprosy have normal or hyperactive antibody production and may produce excessive amounts of autoantibodies. They may even have false-positive VDRL and LE cell tests. They may produce antibodies to a variety of their own tissues. This autoimmune feature is similar in some respects to that seen in the collagen-vascular diseases.

Herpes

Much has been written about the immunology of herpes simplex infections and a comprehensive discussion of this important virus is beyond the scope of this chapter. Suffice it to say that herpes simplex remains latent in neural tissues and can cause active disease when the immune system is suppressed. Many exogenous factors suppress cellular immunity and lead to a recurrence of herpes simplex. These so called "triggers" include fever, ultraviolet light, corticosteroids, and stress. Antibody formation occurs regularly in herpes simplex infection, however, it is generally believed that most types of antiviral antibody do not control the proliferation of herpesvirus.

Cellular immunity appears to be the crucial immunologic mechanism for preventing recurrent attacks of herpes.[13] Profound uveal inflammation can be associated with longstanding herpetic corneal disease. It is not clear whether herpes uveitis represents a direct infection of the uveal tract with virus or whether hypersensitivity mechanisms are responsible. It has been suggested that the virus can alter host tissues and provoke an autoimmune response against ocular tissue which appears foreign to the immune system. Attempts to treat herpes simplex infections with immunopotentiators, or substances that augment the immune response, make sense theoretically but have been disappointing in practice.

Herpes zoster is another neurotropic virus that has an affinity for the skin and the eye. It is interesting that this virus, which is responsible for both chickenpox and shingles, can have such different clinical manifestations in children and adults. It may be that chickenpox is the clinical picture that develops in the immunologically naive host, while shingles develops in a host with partial immunity. It is well established that most adults who develop herpes zoster have some temporary or permanent suppression of cellular immunity.[14] This may be related to aging, malignancy, immunosuppressive therapy, chronic illness, or trauma. It has been demonstrated that varicella can be prevented by passive immunization with antibody to VZ virus. The role of antibody in prevention of herpes zoster, however, and the eventual recovery from both zoster and varicella are somewhat less clear.

Rubella

The rubella virus produces a devastating syndrome of fetal malformations involving the eye, heart, and ear. Ocular defects are seen in 30% to 60% of infants exposed to rubella *in utero,* the most frequent being cataracts and retinopathy. The reason for the persistence of the virus in the fetus is not understood. Maternal IgG antibody crosses the placenta and IgM antibody is produced by the fetus. However, at this early stage of development, cellular immunity is depressed, and this may be related to the inability to clear the virus from fetal tissues.[15]

Cytomegalovirus

Cytomegalovirus produces a chronic infection in newborns and in immunosuppressed adults. It is also a common complication of the acquired immunodeficiency syndrome (AIDS). The virus has been detected in up to 90% of kidney transplant recipients. Cytomegalovirus infection is closely associated with suppression of both cellular and humoral immunity.[16] The mechanism is not fully understood, but it has been suggested that viral infections of antibody producing cells may divert lymphoid cells from their normal immune function and toward producing more virus. Ocular involvement is characterized by focal necrotizing retinochoroiditis and intraretinal hemorrhages.

Candida

Candida albicans is a ubiquitous fungus that produces systemic disease and ocular complications in immunologically compromised individuals. Candida infections occur in patients with diabetes mellitus or neoplasms, in those receiving intravenous hyperalimentation, and in intravenous drug abusers. Both humoral and cellular immunity collaborate to defend the host against candidal infection. Patients with chronic mucocutaneous candidiasis have defects in cellular immunity that apparently lead to chronic candidal infection. These patients develop superficial infection of the nails, skin, and mucous membranes. Candida also tends to proliferate in patients who are receiving corticosteroids or immunosuppressive therapy. Ocular manifestations include cottony whitish lesions of the retina and cellular aggregates in the vitreous. Retinal hemorrhages may also be seen.

Histoplasmosis

Histoplasmosis is caused by the dimorphic fungus *Histoplasma capsulatum*. The disease is common in certain parts of the country, especially the Midwest, and many individuals have asymptomatic and inactive pulmonary lesions. The ocular counterpart of this infection, presumed ocular histoplasmosis, is characterized by peripheral atrophic scars of the retina and choroid. These scars are thought to be secondary to hematogenous dissemination of the organisms. It is not clear when these lesions develop; however, choroiditis must be so mild that lesions are almost never recognized in their active stage.

Cellular immunity is important in the recovery from histoplasmosis infection.[17] Patients who have been exposed to the fungus have strongly positive delayed hypersensitivity skin tests and positive antibody tests. In widespread infection, the immune response may be so depressed that antibody and cellular immunity are not detectable by conventional methods. Individuals with presumed ocular histoplasmosis usually have intact immune responses. Histoplasmosis is another example of an infection that usually is mild and often asymptomatic. Rarely, the infection becomes disseminated and overwhelms the immune system. Perhaps individuals who acquire histoplasmosis are temporarily immunosuppressed or perhaps they are genetically vulnerable to this usually benign infection.

Autoimmune Causes of Uveitis

Autoimmune diseases are those in which an individual develops an inflammatory response against his own tissues. This is essentially the same type of response that is mounted against foreign antigens. It is as though the immune system perceives the host's own tissues as foreign rather than "self." The most familiar autoimmune diseases are the collagen-vascular diseases: rheumatoid arthritis, systemic lupus erythematosus, and polyarteritis nodosa. Interestingly, the incidence of uveitis is probably no higher among patients with these systemic immunologic diseases than it is among the general population.

The autoimmune diseases that most often affect the uvea are those associated with genetic markers on the surface of ocular cells and most other nucleated cells. The markers that have been best studied are those of the HLA system, so named because they were first identified on human leukocytes. Anterior uveitis is commonly associated with HLA-B27. Patients with Behçet's disease have a high incidence HLA-B5, and patients with birdshot choroidopathy have a high incidence of HLA-A29. It is not known at the present time whether the HLA antigens themselves are targets of the immune system, whether the genes for these markers are closely linked to abnormal immune response genes, or whether individuals with these markers are susceptible to microorganisms that produce uveitis.

There has been considerable interest in the role of immune complexes in the development of uveitis. Immune complexes are formed by a combination of antigen and antibody. They precipitate in joints, blood vessels, and in other tissues. When immune complexes are deposited, inflammatory cells are attracted to the area with resultant tissue damage. Many types of vasculitis and arthritis appear to be immune complex-mediated, and it seems probable that immune complexes are trapped in the uveal tract in certain types of uveitis. It is also believed that vasculitis accompanying chronic cyclitis, sarcoid, and Behçet's disease may have an immune complex basis.

Retinal S-antigen is a substance that can be isolated from the retinal photoreceptor region of several animals. Immunization with S-antigen leads to an experimental autoimmune uveitis and circulating lymphocytes from some uveitis patients undergo transformation in the presence of S-antigen. It has been suggested that S-antigen may be a "sequestered" substance that can be recognized by the immune system only after damage to uveoretinal tissue. Once uncovered, the immune system may attack the uvea and retina as though it were foreign tissue. It is possible that S-antigen and other sequestered antigens play a role in certain kinds of autoimmune uveitis.

Ankylosing Spondylitis and Reiter's Syndrome

Over 90% of patients with ankylosing spondylitis are positive for HLA-B27 and approximately 25% develop iridocyclitis.[18] This represents the highest association between an HLA type and a disease entity. Over 90% of patients with Reiter's syndrome have HLA-B27. Chlamydia, mycoplasma, and shigella have all been irregularly associated with Reiter's syndrome.

Juvenile Rheumatoid Arthritis

Patients with juvenile rheumatoid arthritis (JRA) have a high incidence of iridocyclitis. Antinuclear antibodies are found in 88% of JRA patients with iridocyclitis and antinuclear antibodies may be predictive for the development of iridocylitis.[19] An infectious etiology has also been suggested for JRA, but so far, there is no conclusive evidence for this.

Chronic Cyclitis

Some patients with chronic cyclitis (pars planitis, peripheral uveitis) are markedly sensitive to streptococcal antigens. The retinal vasculitis that sometimes accompanies this disease suggests an immune complex deposition in the ciliary body. Circulating immune complexes have been detected in over 60% of patients with chronic cyclitis, and these levels can be correlated with increased disease activity.[20]

Sarcoidosis

Sarcoidosis is a multisystem disease of unknown etiology that affects the lungs, lymph nodes, and eyes. Ocular findings occur in about 25% of cases. A striking feature is the well-known skin test anergy, a failure of response to common skin test antigens such as mumps and candida.[21] Corresponding defects in lymphocyte function can be uncovered with *in vitro* testing. Aside from the depression of delayed hypersensitivity, proliferation of lymphoid tissue is quite common, and high levels of immunoglobulins may be produced.

Sympathetic Ophthalmia

The immunologic aspects of sympathetic ophthalmia have probably been more widely studied than those of almost any other ocular disease. The concept that an injury to the uveal tract could immunize the victim and lead to an attack on the uninjured eye makes this disease an attractive model for the investigation of autoimmune phenomena. In fact, it has not been easy to establish the immunopathogenesis of sympathetic ophthalmia, and it remains unclear which antigen and which effector mechanism are important in this disease. Antibodies and lymphocytes directed against uveal tissue have been demonstrated in sympathetic ophthalmia patients.[22] But it remains unclear whether the immunologic findings in sympathetic ophthalmia are the cause or the effect of uveal injury. Owing to the rarity of sympathetic ophthalmia, it is unlikely that the immunologic events that lead to inflammation of the uninjured eye will be revealed in the near future.

Behçet's Disease

Behçet's disease is a chronic inflammatory condition with widespread clinical manifestations. Among these are iritis, recurrent oral and genital ulcers, vasculitis, arthritis, and skin lesions. Behçet was the first to propose a viral etiology for this disease and this possibility has not been eliminated. Autoantibodies to oral mucosa and lymphocytes which transform in the presence of mucosal antigens are found in Behçet's disease patients.[23] HLA-B5 has been associated with Behçet's disease, especially in Japan. Immunoglobulins and complement are deposited in blood vessel walls. While none of these findings are proof of an immunologic etiology, at least they demonstrate that the immune system is active in this condition.

Vogt-Koyanagi-Harada Syndrome

Vogt-Koyanagi-Harada syndrome (VKH) is a multisystem disease affecting the eye, the skin, and the central nervous system. Antibodies to uveal pigment and melanin have been detected in patients with VKH, and this may explain the uveal depigmentation and vitiligo associated with this condition. Heightened cellular and humoral immunity to uveal antigens have been demonstrated and a decreased number of peripheral blood lymphocytes have been noted.[24]

Lens-Induced Uveitis

Very strong organ-specific antigens have been found in the lens. They may be sequestered antigens, similar to S-antigen, and it has been suggested that uncovering these lens antigens through injury may allow the immune system to react to the unfamiliar protein. Heightened cellular and humoral immunity to lens protein has been found in lens-induced uveitis.[25] The rarity of this condition makes systematic investigation of lens-induced uveitis very difficult.

Recurrence of Uveitis

It seems reasonable to speculate that the recurrent nature of uveitis may be linked to some type of immunologic mechanism, but we are a long way from having a clear understanding of this mechanism. O'Connor has suggested that certain causal factors in uveitis should be analyzed in an attempt to explain its recurrent nature.[26]

Latent Organisms

Good evidence exists for latency of herpes simplex virus and toxoplasma in ocular tissues. Periodic release of these organisms is probably associated with recurrent uveal inflammation. Herpes simplex virus can remain latent in ganglia for many years, periodically traveling down sensory or sympathetic nerve axons to repopulate an area of corneal epithelium and causing a recurrent lesion in that tissue. Toxoplasma cysts may break down periodically, allowing organisms to affect local retinal tissue. It has been suggested that specific antibody or cellular immunity is responsible for maintaining the intactness of the cyst, and that periodic lapses in immunity may permit the toxoplasma organisms to come out of their cysts.

Pregnancy

A number of hormonal changes occur during pregnancy including increased levels of estrogen and endogenous corticosteroids. Increased numbers of suppressor lymphocytes induce a state of tolerance that allows acceptance of the fetus. There seems to be an increased susceptibility to toxoplasma infection during pregnancy, possibly due to hormonal or immunologic alterations. However, it is now well established that a woman with recurrent ocular toxoplasmosis during pregnancy will not transmit the infection to her fetus, nor in most cases will she succumb to generalized infection with toxoplasma.

Aging Changes

Cellular immunity generally declines with age, and this may be a factor in the recurrence of uveitis in the elderly. This is particularly likely with ocular toxoplasmosis and herpes zoster. On the other hand, one could postulate that exuberant cellular and humoral responses, which play a role in recurrent uveitis in younger patients, will wane with the aging process.

Changes in Permeability

Damage to uveal vasculature or to epithelial barriers of the uveal tract may cause long-lasting changes in permeability. This altered structure may favor the deposition of immune complexes or may facilitate the passage of inflammatory cells in some other way.

Emotional Stress

It has long been observed that emotional stress can precipitate a variety of disease states, including uveitis. Much progress has been made in sorting out the neurophysiologic connections, hormonal release, and immunologic changes caused by emotional stress. Recently, it has been recognized that stress causes release of endorphins in the central nervous system, and it appears that some of the effects of stress are mediated through the release of substance P, a neuropeptide found in certain neurons of the ventral brain stem. When released at nerve terminals, substance P causes degranulation of mast cells and activators of macrophages. The hypothalamus is believed to play an extremely important role in stress-mediated inflammatory reactions. A better understanding of the role of neurotransmitters and the autonomic nervous system may be important to our understanding of the factors that lead to the recurrence of uveitis.

Modulation of the Immune Response

Some of the most convincing evidence of an immunologic basis for uveitis is the dramatic response of many types of uveal inflammation to corticosteroids and other agents that suppress the immune response. Corticosteroids have long been the mainstay of treatment in uveitis. They are effective both topically and systemically. Corticosteroids appear to work by a redistribution of blood lymphocytes and other leukocytes in the vascular compartment and by a variety of effects on the function of cells in the circulation and in tissues.[27]

Antimetabolite drugs interfere with the synthesis of nucleic acid or protein or both. These agents are quite potent and have extensive toxic effects. They are not generally the first line drugs for uveitis; however, when corticosteroids fail to control uveal inflammation, a course of antimetabolite therapy is often recommended. Cyclosporine has potent immunosuppressive actions with specific anti-T cell effects. This effect may be due to cyclosporine's influence on interleukin-2, a soluble product of activated helper T cells. Encouraging results with cyclosporine have been obtained in certain refractory cases of uveitis. However, nephrotoxicity and an increased incidence of lymphoma with cyclosporine suggest that the enthusiasm for this drug must be tempered with the same concerns that have restricted the use of other immunosuppressives.

Because of the many side-effects of corticosteroids and antimetabolites, ophthalmologists have long been interested in nonsteroidal anti-inflammatory agents. While these agents have been reasonably effective in the control of scleritis and episcleritis, they have been notably ineffective in the treatment of uveitis. As we learn more about the pathways of arachidonic acid metabolism, it may become possible to select nonsteroidal agents that can more effectively control the mediators of uveal inflammation.

Even though the thrust of uveitis treatment is toward down-regulation of the immune response, in certain types of uveitis, a case can be made for the use of immunopotentiators, agents that enhance the immune response. Such agents could possibly overcome persistent or latent infections by boosting certain elements of the immune system, such as helper T cells, macrophages, or B cells, and remove unwanted antigens from the eye. Such was the hope with levamisol and interferon, but so far, the available evidence has not encouraged the intensive study of these agents for uveitis treatment.

It seems apparent that the immune system plays a major role in the initiation, recurrence, and eventual resolution of uveitis. As we learn more about the immune system, the mechanisms which cause uveal inflammation may become even more complex than we now imagine. As we unravel the pathways of uveal inflammation and the immune system, we hope to gain insight into the pathogenesis and the treatment of uveitis.

References

1. Waksman BH, Bullington SJ: Studies of arthritis and other lesions induced in rats by injection of mycobacterial adjuvants. III. Lesions of the eye. Arch Ophthalmol 64:751, 1960
2. Friedlaender MH, Krasnobrod H: Ocular findings in systemic cutaneous basophil hypersensitivity. Invest Ophthalmol Vis Sci 18:964–969, 1979
3. Smelser GK, Silver S: The distribution of mast cells in the normal eye: A method of study. Exp Eye Res 2:134, 1963
4. Friedlaender MH, Howes EL, Hall J et al: Morphology of delayed hypersensitivity in the uveal tract. Invest Ophthalmol Vis Sci 17:327, 1978
5. Friedlaender MH, Dvorak HF: Morphology of delayed type hypersensitivity reactions in the guinea pig cornea. J Immunol 118:1558, 1977
6. Austen KF: Tissue mast cells in immediate hypersensitivity. In Dixon FJ, Fisher DW, (eds): The Biology of Immunologic Disease pp 223–233. Sunderland, MD, Sinauer, 1984
7. Parker J, Goetzl EJ, Friedlaender MH: Leukotrienes in the aqueous humor of patients with uveitis. Arch Ophthalmol 104:722, 1986
8. Frigas E, Gleich GJ: The eosinophil and the pathophysiology of asthma. J Allergy Clin Immunol 77:527–537, 1986
9. Perkins ES: Ocular toxoplasmosis. Br J Ophthalmol 57:1, 1973
10. Brown DH: Ocular toxocara. II. Clinical review. J Exp Med 141:483, 1975
11. Kaplan BS, Wigelsworth FW, Marks ML et al: The glomerulopathy of congenital syphilis—An immune complex disease. J Pediatr 81:1154, 1972
12. Waldorf DS, Sheagren JN, Trautman JR et al: Impaired delayed hypersensitivity in patients with lepromatous leprosy. Lancet 2:773, 1966
13. Easty DL, Maini RN, Jones BR: Cellular immunity in herpes simplex keratitis. Trans Ophthalmol Soc UK 93:171, 1973

14. Morisson WL: Viral warts, herpes simplex and herpes zoster in patients with secondary immune deficiencies and neoplasms. Br J Dermatol 92:625, 1975
15. White LR, Leikin S, Villavicencio O et al: Immune competency in congenital rubella: Lymphocyte transformation, delayed hypersensitivity, and response to vaccination. J Pediatr 73:229, 1968
16. Kantor GL, Goldberg LS, Johnson BM et al: Immunologic abnormalities induced by post-perfusion cytomegalovirus infection. Ann Intern Med 73:533, 1970
17. Ganley JP: The role of the cellular immune system in patients with macular disciform histoplasmosis. Int Ophthalmol Clin 15:83, 1975
18. Brewerton DA, Caffrey M, Hart FD et al: Ankylosing Spondylitis and HL-A27. Lancet 1:904, 1973
19. Schaller JG, Johnson GD, Holborow EJ et al: The association of antinuclear antibodies with chronic iridocyclitis of juvenile rheumatoid arthritis (Still's Disease). Arth Rheum 17:409, 1974
20. Char DH, Stein P, Masi R et al: Immune complexes and uveitis. Am J Ophthalmol 87:678, 1979
21. James DG, Neville E, Walker A: Immunology of sarcoidosis. Am J Med 59:388, 1975
22. Wong VG, Anderson R, O'Brien PJ: Sympathetic ophthalmia and lymphocyte transformation. Am J Ophthalmol 72:960, 1971
23. Oshima Y, Shimizu T, Yokohari R et al: Clinical studies on Behçet's Syndrome. Ann Rheum Dis 22:36, 1963
24. Hammer H: Cellular hypersensitivity to uveal pigment in sympathetic ophthalmia and Vogt-Koyanagi-Harada Syndrome. Br J Ophthalmol 55:850, 1971
25. Rahi AHS, Misra RN, Morgan G: Immunopathology of the lens. III. Humoral and cellular immune responses to autologous lens antigens and their roles in ocular inflammation. Br J Ophthalmol 61:371, 1977
26. O'Connor GR: Factors related to the initiation and recurrence of uveitis. Am J Ophthalmol 96:577, 1983
27. Friedlaender MH: Corticosteroid therapy of ocular inflammation. Int Ophthalmol Clin 23:175, 1983

FOUR

Corneal Disease and Surgery Associated With Uveitis

Many conditions that affect the uveal tract also affect the cornea. The cornea and uveal tract may be separate targets of a disease process, or these tissues may be simultaneously inflamed because of their contiguity. Keratouveitis may be part of a very specific syndrome or it may be rather nonspecific. In this chapter, we will consider a wide spectrum of keratouveitis, the diagnostic value of sampling the cornea in uveitis, and the treatment of a wide spectrum of keratouveitis syndromes.

Nonspecific Corneal Changes in Uveitis

There are several nonspecific manifestations of uveitis such as cell and flare in the anterior chamber, iris hyperemia, and vasculitis. Some nonspecific changes affect the cornea. The most obvious is keratic precipitates, which are collections of mononuclear cells on the corneal endothelium. Both lymphocytes and macrophages have been identified as components of keratic precipitates. They may be distributed randomly over the entire endothelial surface, or they may be localized to a smaller central or inferior region. In Fuchs' heterochromic iridocyclitis, we see small white keratic precipitates distributed over the entire endothelial surface. This arrangement is quite characteristic of Fuchs' uveitis and is helpful in making the diagnosis.[1] In contrast, the keratic precipitates of herpes simplex keratouveitis

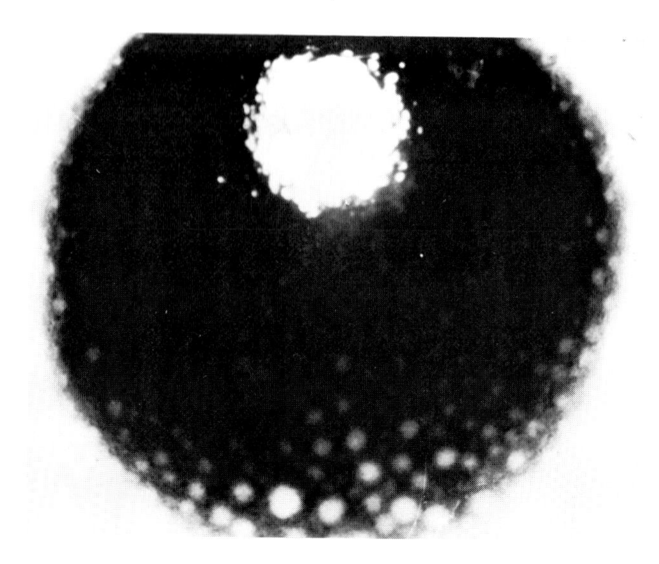

Figure 4-1. Mutton fat keratic precipitates in sarcoid uveitis.

are usually located directly behind the area of corneal stromal inflammation. This distribution suggests that inflammatory cells are attracted to a very precise inflammatory focus within the cornea. Mutton fat keratic precipitates (Fig. 4-1) are large, greasy endothelial deposits, found in granulomatous types of inflammation, such as sarcoid, tuberculosis, and syphilis. Their cellular composition is largely mononuclear. In most other types of uveitis, keratic precipitates are localized centrally and inferiorly. Presumably, the inferior location is due to convection currents within the anterior chamber.

Corneal edema is rarely observed in severe uveitis.[2] Endotheleitis may lead to temporary or permanent endothelial dysfunction and inhibition of aqueous humor by the cornea. Surprisingly often, the corneal endothelium recovers and edema ultimately disappears. Rarely, permanent endothelial decompensation related to uveitis may occur. Apparently, the corneal endothelium can withstand severe and prolonged inflammatory insults.

Both high and low intra-ocular pressure can lead to corneal edema. With high intra-ocular pressures, epithelial edema develops first. Small epithelial vesicles may form, and when they coalesce, larger bullae may form. High and long-standing pressure elevation leads to stromal edema. A thickened corneal stroma with folds in Descemet's membrane suggests a more serious type of dysfunction.

Stromal edema is also seen in hypotensive ocular conditions. This type of edema is not due to endothelial dysfunction but rather to a lack of compressive forces from within the eye. In such cases, stromal edema disappears when normal intraocular pressure is restored.

Band keratopathy (Fig. 4-2) is a deposition of calcium in the cornea. It develops in many types of uveitis, particularly those that are chronic and those that occur early in life.[3] Band keratopathy is often seen in the uveitis that accom-

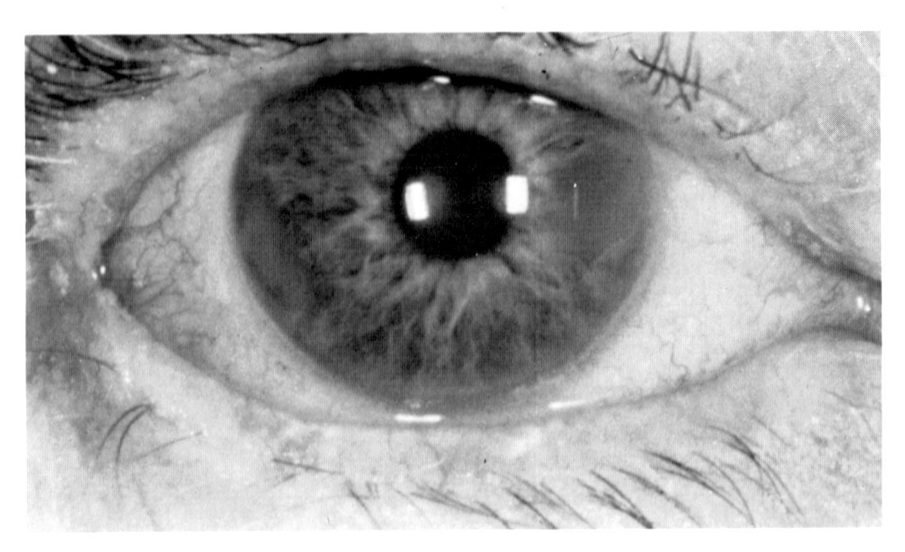

Figure 4-2. Early calcific band keratopathy.

panies juvenile rheumatoid arthritis; however, it may be seen in other types of chronic uveitis. Many systemic diseases, especially those in which calcium is mobilized, are accompanied by band keratopathy.

Microscopically, calcium deposition begins in the region of Bowman's layer (Fig. 4-3). The epithelium and stroma may be affected as deposition continues. Clinically, deposition is usually confined to the interpalpebral region. The periph-

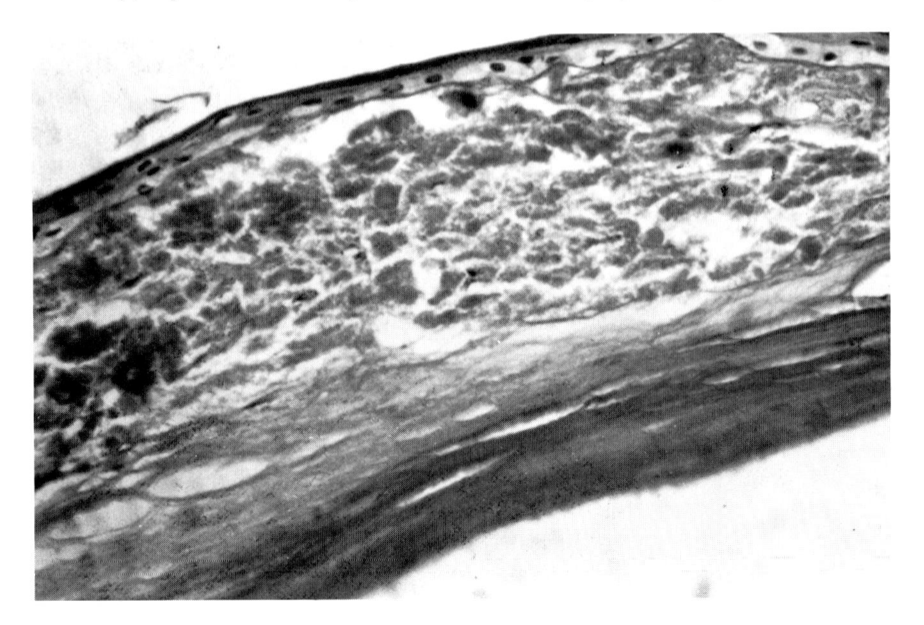

Figure 4-3. Calcium deposition in Bowman's layer of the cornea.

eral cornea is affected first, although there is usually a clear zone between the band and the limbus. In time, the central cornea is affected. One can usually see tiny (Swiss cheese) holes throughout the band. These correspond to gaps in Bowman's layer where corneal nerves enter the epithelium from the stroma.

The reason for calcific band formation in uveitis and other conditions is unknown. It has been suggested that evaporation of water from the interpalpebral region leads to a localized elevation of *p*H that favors the deposition of calcium. Whatever the pathogenesis, the deposition of calcium in the central cornea can lead to profound loss of vision and sometimes permanent corneal scarring. Much of the calcium can be removed by chelation; this will be discussed in more detail in a later section.

Keratouveitis Syndromes

We can divide keratouveitis syndromes into three categories: infectious, noninfectious, and mechanical. The infectious causes are associated with a wide variety of microorganisms: bacterial, viral, fungal, and parasitic. The noninfectious causes are usually attributed to autoimmune diseases. The mechanical causes include trauma, medications, chemicals, and surgery.

Infectious Keratouveitis

Corneal infections are usually associated with some degree of uveal inflammation. The uveitis may be minimal or profound. The extent of uveal inflammation depends on the etiologic agent and the duration of the infection. Bacteria such as *Staphylococcus aureus, Streptococcus pneumoniae,* and *Pseudomonas aeruginosa* are highly pyogenic and are often associated with intense anterior chamber reactions. It is not unusual to find a hypopyon in acute bacterial keratitis (Fig. 4-4). Many opportunistic organisms produce an indolent keratitis and are associated with low-grade anterior chamber reaction. This group includes organisms such as *Staphylococcus epidermidis, Streptococcus viridans,* and *Moraxella liquifaciens.* The corneal infiltrate usually precedes the anterior chamber reaction and, in general, the larger, deeper, and more long-standing the keratitis, the more profound the anterior chamber reaction.

Fungal keratitis may also be associated with uveitis and keratic precipitates. Since fungal keratitis is usually indolent, the anterior chamber reaction is usually mild. However, in long-standing fungal keratitis, a severe anterior chamber reaction and hypopyon formation might be expected. Filamentous fungi are typically associated with corneal trauma in previously healthy eyes. On the other hand, yeast infections develop in eyes with pre-existing corneal disease.[4] Candida frequently occurs in the hospital environment, especially in the immunocompromised host. Fusarium is associated with trauma, especially from vegetable matter.

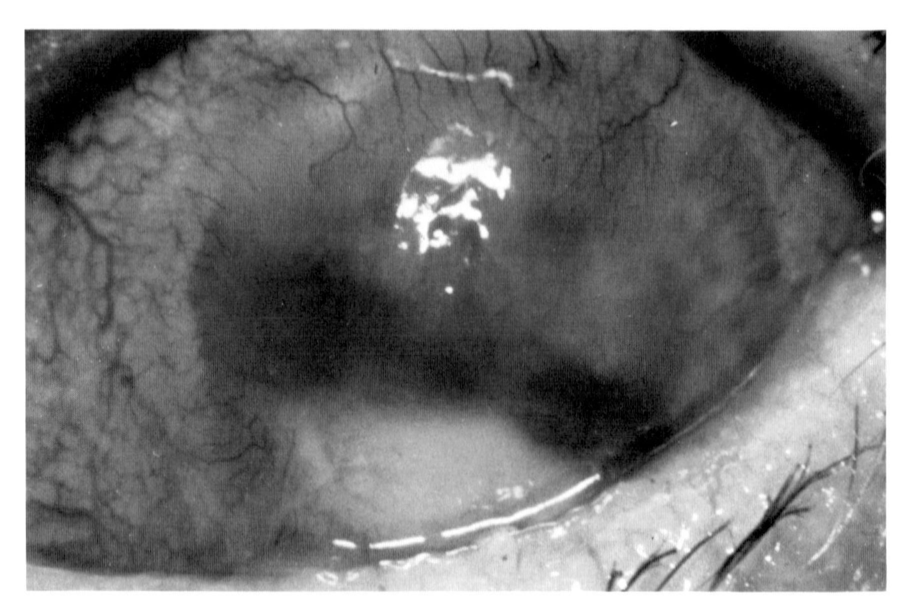

Figure 4-4. Bacterial keratitis with hypopyon.

Parasitic infections are not frequently encountered in the United States. However, *Onchocerca volvulus* is a common cause of keratouveitis in sub-Saharan Africa and in certain parts of South America.[5] In these locations, whole villages may be blind from the disease known as "river blindness." The organism is transmitted to man by the Black Simulian fly, which breeds near river beds. Affected individuals develop subcutaneous nodules and have blood-borne dissemination of the microfilaria. These microfilaria can lodge in the eye and can be visualized in the cornea and anterior chamber. A low-grade keratitis and anterior chamber reaction accompany the infection (Fig. 4-5).

A recently recognized cause of parasitic keratouveitis is acanthamoeba.[6] This parasite is being seen with increasing frequency among contact lens wearers (Fig. 4-6). Poor hygiene and use of nonsterile distilled water appear to be factors in the alarming rise of this infection.

Endophthalmitis can affect the cornea secondarily when intra-ocular infection cannot be controlled. Infiltration of the endothelial surface of the cornea occurs. As the infection progresses, the entire stroma may be affected. Organisms can sometimes be cultured from the corneal stroma. Fortunately, uncontrolled endophthalmitis is rare due to improved diagnostic techniques such as vitreous biopsy and therapeutic techniques such as vitrectomy.[7]

Herpes simplex keratouveitis (Fig. 4-7) is one of the most common causes of keratouveitis in ophthalmic practice. The corneal infection can take several forms: dendritic keratitis, disciform edema, or interstitial keratitis. The uveal tract is involved secondarily. A few cells in the anterior chamber may be detected

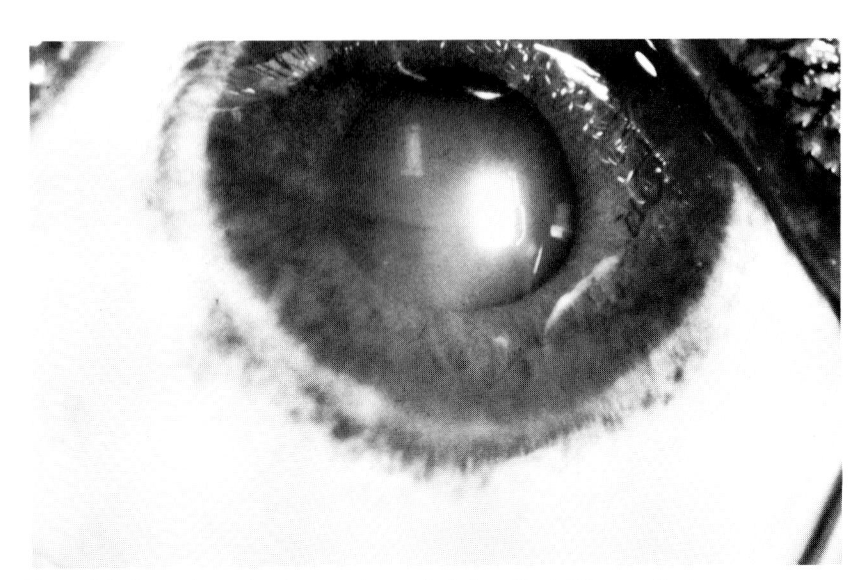

Figure 4-5. Corneal scarring from onchocerciasis in a West African patient.

in dendritic keratitis. With stromal involvement, keratic precipitates accumulate behind the affected cornea. With interstitial keratitis, the anterior chamber reaction is much more intense and hypopyon formation may occur. More intense reactions appear to be related to stromal inflammation and necrosis, a process

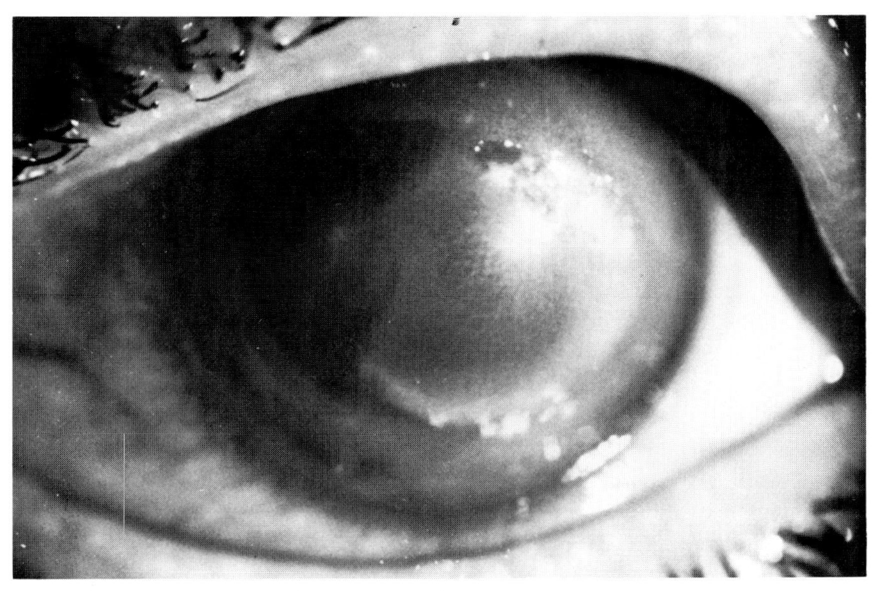

Figure 4-6. *Acanthamoeba* keratitis in a contact lens wearer.

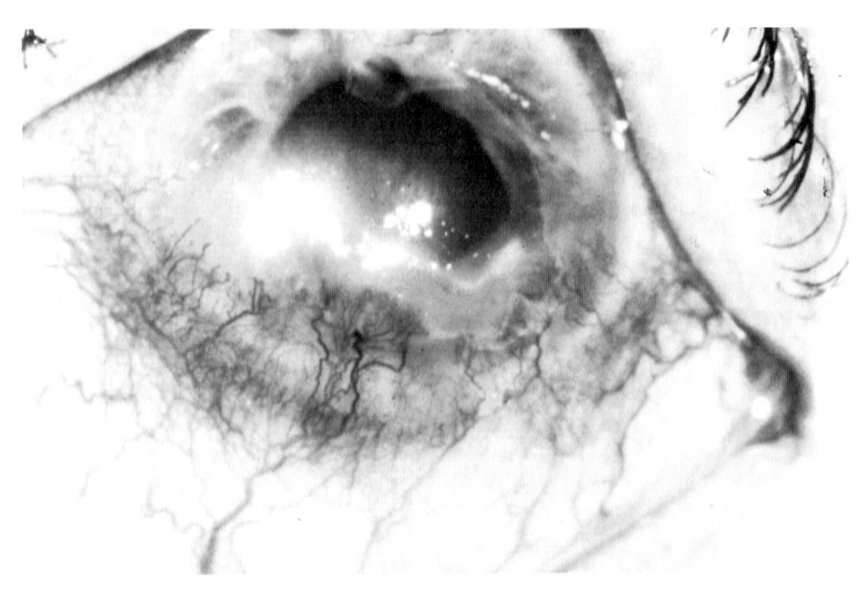

Figure 4-7. Severe herpes simplex keratouveitis.

in which chemotactic factors and many other mediators of inflammation are liberated.

Herpes zoster keratouveitis (Fig. 4-8) is characterized by a deeper and frequently more intense ocular inflammation than herpes simplex.[8] While dendritic

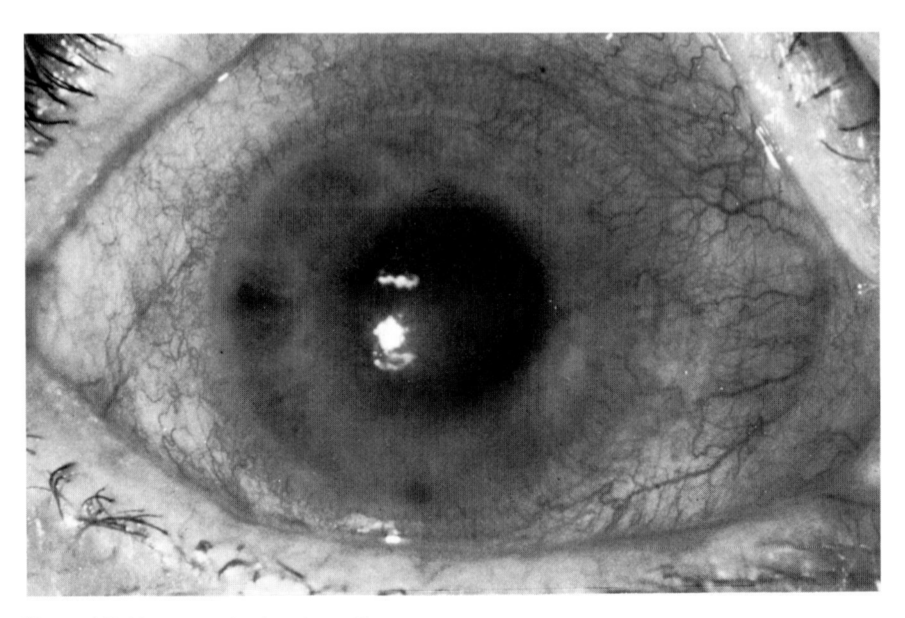

Figure 4-8. Herpes zoster keratouveitis.

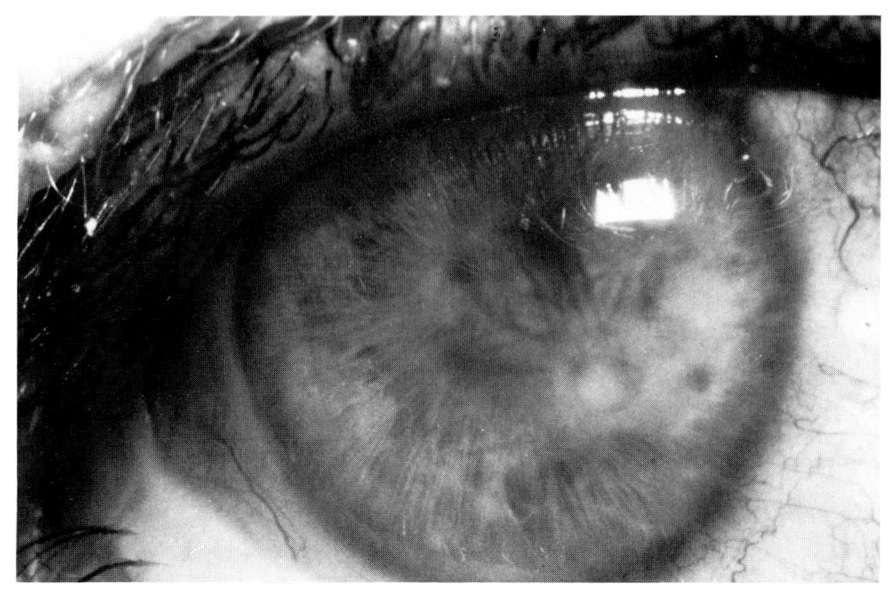

Figure 4-9. Corneal scarring from presumed luetic interstitial keratitis.

epithelial lesions are sometimes observed, the typical zoster infection consists of stromal keratitis and uveitis. Corneal scarring and vascularization are common sequelae of the corneal inflammation. Iris atrophy and depigmentation are also common. Ocular involvement occurs when the nasociliary branch of the ophthalmic division of the trigeminal nerve is affected. Skin lesions in the distribution of the ophthalmic nerve are almost always present.

Congenital syphilis is often associated with interstitial keratitis. The onset of the disease is between the ages of 5 and 15 years. Stromal infiltration and opacification are seen (Fig. 4-9). Low-grade iritis is seen when the keratitis is active, and the reaction subsides as the disease becomes quiescent. Interstitial keratitis probably represents an immunologic inflammation of the cornea rather than a direct corneal infection.

Mycobacterial keratitis (Fig. 4-10) is uncommon, but it is another form of indolent corneal inflammation that must be kept in mind. Diagnosis is often difficult since acid-fast stains are not done routinely. In addition, mycobacteria may be highly refractory to antibiotic therapy. Many reported cases have required excisional keratoplasty.[9]

Noninfectious Keratouveitis

Noninfectious forms of keratouveitis are usually attributed to immunologic mechanisms. In some conditions, such as rheumatoid arthritis, the immunologic events are fairly well defined. But in Mooren's ulcer, a severe, debilitating form of peripheral keratitis, the immunologic events are obscure.

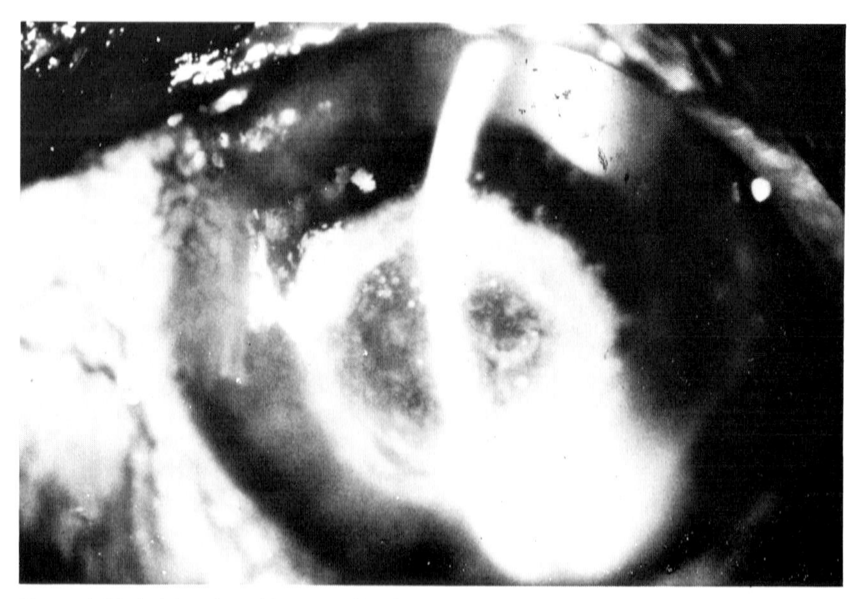

Figure 4-10. Indolent keratitis caused by *Mycobacteria chelonei.*

Sarcoid has many hallmarks of an infectious disease, yet attempts to isolate an infectious agent have been unsuccessful. Sarcoid is characterized by granulomatous inflammation and can affect many different tissues of the eye. Most prominently, sarcoid produces a panuveitis involving the iris, choroid, and ciliary body. Retinal vasculitis, snowball opacities in the vitreous, and candlewax exudates on the retina are frequently present. Koeppe nodules may be seen on the iris, and mutton fat keratic precipitates may occur on the cornea. Aside from keratic precipitates, corneal signs of sarcoid have not been given much attention. Recently, however, a prismatic effect of the inferior peripheral cornea has been noted in patients with sarcoid uveitis.[10] This effect seems to be due to thickening of the inferior peripheral cornea. The prismatic effect is probably a nonspecific sign, but it is striking how often it is associated with sarcoid uveitis. It may represent an accumulation of keratic precipitates along the inferior cornea and corneal swelling related to endothelial dysfunction.

The ocular findings in sarcoid may be quite subtle, especially in white patients. For this reason, the presence of the prismatic effect can alert the ophthalmologist to the possibility of sarcoid uveitis. When blood tests such as serum lysozyme and angiotensin converting enzyme are also abnormal, a diagnosis of sarcoid can usually be made.

Mooren's ulcer is highly inflammatory and can be associated with uveal inflammation by contiguity. The extent of uveal inflammation depends on the severity of peripheral corneal inflammation. Morbidity associated with Mooren's ulcer is usually due to corneal thinning and subsequent central corneal involvement.

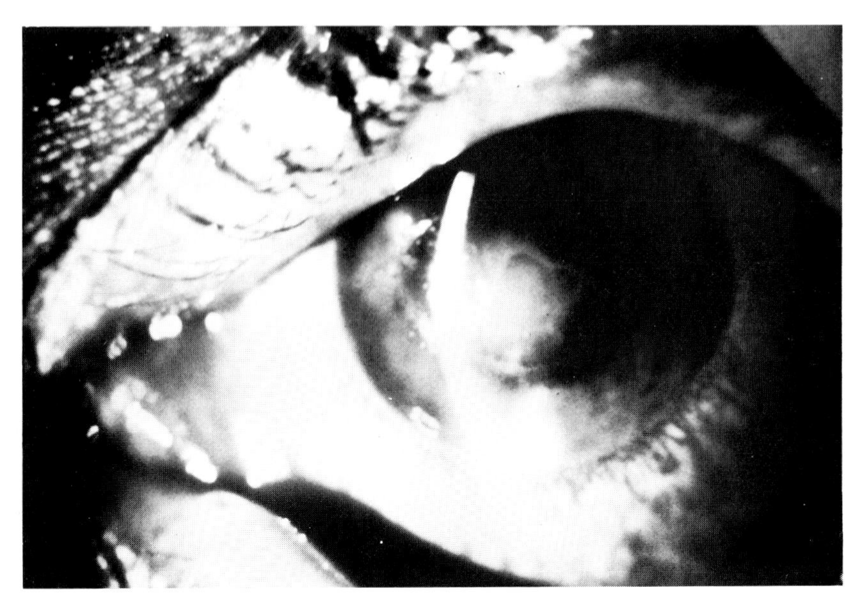

Figure 4-11. Severe toxic keratoconjunctivitis caused by excessive eyedrops.

Rheumatoid arthritis does not have a strong association with uveitis. In fact, the incidence of uveitis among rheumatoid patients is no higher than in the general population. Still, rheumatoid patients develop scleritis and sclerokeratitis and, in these individuals, the uveal tract may be inflamed by contiguity. As in Mooren's ulcer, uveal inflammation is usually mild. Rarely does one observe keratic precipitates or posterior synechiae. In advanced cases, corneal pacification may obscure the view of the anterior chamber, and it may be difficult to assess uveal involvement.

Mechanical Keratouveitis

Corneal abrasions are associated with a small amount of cell and flare in the anterior chamber. Larger abrasions are accompanied by even more reaction. The mechanism is presumably an axonal reflex. The abrasion may be accompanied by spasm of the iris sphincter and the ciliary body. Treatment with cycloplegics reduces or eliminates the spasm, and the anterior chamber reaction dissipates within a few days.

Toxic keratouveitis (Fig. 4-11) can be caused by chemicals or medication. This type of injury may be unintentional, as with alkali burns, or iatrogenic, as with excessive medication. Chemical burns caused by alkali and acid are accompanied by massive uveitis. In these injuries, a direct, corrosive effect of the chemical liberates cells and proteins from the vessels of the anterior segment. Sometimes a hypopyon will form. Usually the anterior chamber reaction is eclipsed by the severe corneal changes that occur in these disastrous injuries.

Toxic keratouveitis can occur with excessive ocular medication in the form of eyedrops and ointments. These are usually cases in which medications have been used frequently for many weeks, months, or even years. Punctate epithelial changes are invariably present, and these lesions may coalesce to form larger epithelial defects. In time, corneal vascularization can develop. The anterior chamber reaction is usually mild or moderate. The mechanism is presumably the same as that seen in corneal abrasions. Patients experience severe pain and photophobia. When the medication is stopped, symptoms improve rapidly.

One of the most frequent forms of uveitis encountered by the ophthalmologist is the postsurgical form. Cataract surgery with or without implantation of intra-ocular lenses, corneal transplants, and other types of anterior segment surgery are invariably accompanied by a low-grade, transient iritis. Usually, this results from manipulation of the iris during surgery. With the popularity of the extracapsular procedure, retained cortical material and lens-induced uveitis are being seen with increasing frequency. It is not unusual for lens-induced uveitis to persist for months following incomplete removal of cortical material. Presumably lens material sensitizes the host leading to prolonged anterior segment inflammation. Patients with this type of lens-induced uveitis relate the onset of redness, discomfort, or photophobia to the time of their cataract surgery. Sometimes it is difficult to find the remaining lens material, and often one is surprised that a small remnant of cortex is lodged behind the iris. Gonioscopy is particularly helpful in locating retained cortical material.

Malplacement of a lens implant is another cause of chronic postsurgical uveitis. There may be several reasons for this. Iris capture by the lens haptics may cause chronic irritation of uveal tissue, or the plastic lens material itself may be coated with a solution that is toxic to the eye. An undersized implant may also irritate the iris and cause a low-grade chronic uveitis. It may be necessary to remove lens implants when they are causing iritis. Often they can be replaced with a better fitting lens implant. Especially favored are posterior chamber and flexible anterior chamber lens implants.

Diagnosis

The cornea may provide useful diagnostic information in certain types of keratouveitis. Decreased corneal sensation is found with both herpes simplex and herpes zoster infections. Corneal anesthesia is most notable directly over the corneal lesion, and sensation remains absent for several months or even years.

In the presence of active epithelial disease, corneal scrapings may show syncytial giant cells (Fig. 4-12), and occasionally intranuclear inclusion bodies. Their presence suggests active replicating virus. Corneal scrapings are of considerable value in keratouveitis associated with bacterial and fungal keratitis. In such cases, the cause of uveitis is readily apparent. Corneal biopsy is performed occasionally, especially in the presence of culture negative corneal infiltrates. Such

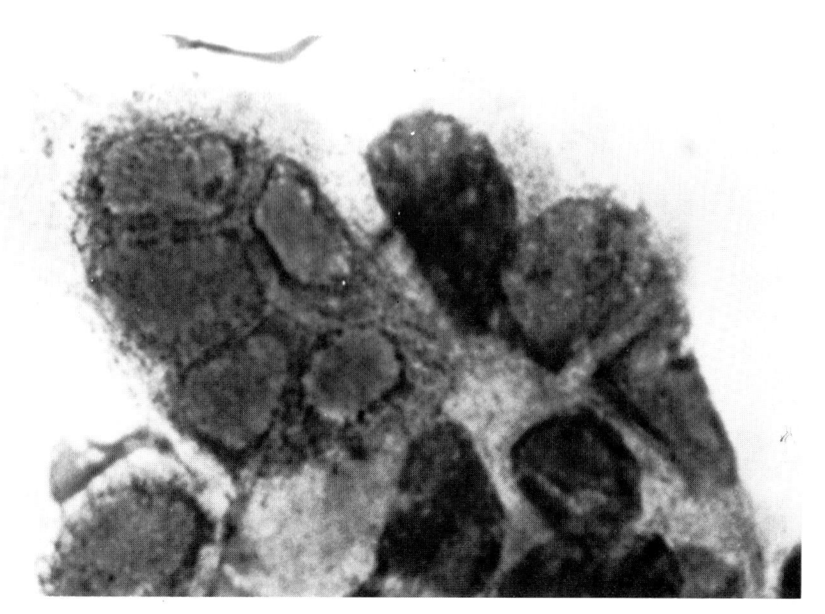

Figure 4-12. Syncytial giant cells in corneal scrapings from a herpes patient.

biopsies are particularly helpful in diagnosing *Acanthamoeba* and mycobacterial keratitis.

Corneal cultures are useful in infectious keratouveitis. Because of the small sample size, it is important to take multiple scrapings from the ulcer bed and smear them directly onto culture plates. We routinely inoculate blood and chocolate agar plates. If a fungal etiology is suspected, Sabouraud's agar is inoculated, and if anaerobic organisms are suspected, thioglycolate and chopped meat broths are inoculated.[11] Löwenstein-Jensen medium is inoculated when mycobacteria are suspected. Acanthamoeba will show optimal growth on non-nutrient agar coated with *Escherichia coli.*

Anterior chamber paracentesis is occasionally used in the diagnosis of keratouveitis. This technique is particularly helpful when infectious endophthalmitis is suspected. Aqueous humor is centrifuged so that the sediment can be examined microscopically and cultured on the appropriate media. The aqueous can also be analyzed for antibody to various organisms, lens material, or uveal pigment. When aqueous humor titers are high with respect to serum titers, it may support a particular kind of uveitis.

Treatment

Nonspecific Corneal Changes

The low-grade iritis that accompanies corneal abrasions is self-limited and requires no treatment in many instances. If severe and if the patient is symptomatic, dilation with mydriatic/cycloplegic drops and patching will help maintain comfort and shorten the course of the iritis. Corticosteroid drops are rarely necessary for traumatic uveitis, and they may be contra-indicated if an infectious process is present. On the other hand, corticosteroids can be helpful in noninfectious causes of uveitis, especially those with an immunologic mechanism. Corticosteroids have a cytolytic effect and help stabilize vascular leakage.[12] They are highly effective in reducing an anterior chamber reaction and keratic precipitates. Their effect may be temporary, and the anterior chamber reaction and keratic precipitates will return if the stimulus for inflammation is not removed.

Corneal edema may be treated with hypertonic saline eyedrops or ointment. The effectiveness of this treatment is often disappointing. If intra-ocular pressure is elevated, glaucoma therapy will be an effective way of reducing corneal edema. If endothelial dysfunction is present, corneal transplantation may be necessary. Bandage contact lenses may occasionally be helpful, especially if the cause of uveitis is a disrupted corneal surface. In such instances, the bandage lens will reduce the surface irritation and allow the anterior segment irritability to subside.

Band keratopathy can be removed by chelation with sodium EDTA. The epithelium overlying the band must first be removed with cocaine, alcohol, or gentle debridement. A 0.37% solution is applied to the cornea. The solution is rubbed into the calcified area and after thorough saturation, the band can be chipped away using a spatula or surgical blade. Care should be taken not to disrupt the anterior stroma so that scarring will be minimal. If EDTA is not available, 0.5% hydrochloric acid or acetic acid may be substituted. After chelation, the pupil should be dilated with atropine, and the eye should be tightly patched until the epithelium heals.

Infectious Keratouveitis

It is crucial to recognize infectious causes of keratouveitis and to treat them with appropriate antimicrobial therapy as soon as possible. Although microbiologic identification will improve the specificity of therapy, it is acceptable and often essential to use broad spectrum therapy until a definite microbiologic diagnosis can be made. Treatment with periocular, topical, or intravitreal antibiotics may be needed.

Occasionally, corneal perforation will occur in the presence of microbial keratitis or mechanical injury. Tissue adhesives have been extremely useful in sealing the cornea and restoring the integrity of the anterior chamber. For larger corneal defects, corneal patch grafts can be cut to the size and shape of the defect. Sometimes, it is more convenient to perform a corneal transplant that encompasses a large corneal defect.

Noninfectious Keratouveitis

Corticosteroids can be used with much greater safety when an infectious condition has been ruled out. Corticosteroids are particularly helpful in sarcoid, collagen-vascular diseases, and postsurgical forms of keratouveitis. It is important to be aware of the side-effects of corticosteroids. Glaucoma and superinfections can occur with a relatively short course of steroid treatment. These complications are less common when systemic steroids are used. However, systemic steroids have their own complications, particularly gastric irritation and bleeding.

Nonsteroidal anti-inflammatory agents have a role in rheumatoid arthritis and other collagen-vascular diseases. Indomethacin and other nonsteroidal agents are useful alternatives to corticosteroids in the treatment of scleritis and sclerokeratitis. Corneal thinning and perforation can occur in noninfectious keratouveitis, particularly when it is associated with a collagen-vascular disease. Scleromalacia perforans is particularly difficult to treat. In such cases, tissue adhesives, patch grafts, and occasionally corneal transplants may be useful.

Mechanical Keratouveitis

Treatment for mild trauma may be unnecessary. The transient iritis associated with a corneal abrasion or corneal foreign body is self-limited and resolves within a few days. Dilation and patching will often speed the resolution of this type of inflammation. When toxic substances are responsible for keratouveitis, their removal will often allow the inflammation to subside. This is particularly true when excessive topical medications are discontinued. A more difficult problem is encountered in the treatment of severe chemical burns due to alkali or acid. These substances often produce a long-standing inflammatory process in which the cornea and anterior segment are irreversibly damaged. Ascorbate, citrate, and topical corticosteroids have been used to treat the inflammation associated with alkali burns.[13] However, when these injuries are severe, treatment is invariably disappointing.

In postoperative uveitis, inflammation is usually transient. It will resolve with time but if quicker resolution is desired, corticosteroids can be used safely. When inflammation is prolonged, one must determine the cause. The first major consideration is whether the inflammation is caused by an infectious or noninfectious process. If an infection is suspected, anterior chamber and vitreous paracentesis must be performed. If infection has been ruled out, one must determine the stimulus for the inflammatory process. Usually it will be due to retained cortex or malposition of a lens implant. Lens cortex can be removed by aspiration under sterile operating room conditions. A malpositioned lens implant can be repositioned or, if necessary, removed.

Conclusion

When evaluating a uveitis patient, the cornea should be examined closely. It may provide clues to the etiology of the uveitis. It should be kept in mind that corneal inflammation may occur either before or after uveal inflammation. Sampling the cornea through scraping, culture, or biopsy may shed light on the etiology of keratouveitis. This is particularly true of infectious conditions. Treating the corneal pathology will frequently allow the keratouveitis to resolve. Treatment of corneal complications will help the overall management of the uveitis patient.

References

1. Kimura SJ: Fuchs' syndrome of heterochromic cyclitis in brown-eyed patients. Trans Am Ophthalmol Soc 76:76–89, 1978
2. Dohlman CH: Physiology of the cornea. In Smolin G, Thoft RA (eds): The Cornea, pp 3–17. Boston, Little Brown & Co, 1983
3. O'Connor GR: Calcific band keratopathy. Trans Am Ophthalmol Soc 70:58, 1952
4. Koenig SB: Fungal keratitis. In Tabbara KF, Hyndiuk RA (eds): Infections of the Eye, pp 331–342. Boston, Little Brown & Co, 1986
5. Garner A: Pathology of ocular onchocerciasis: Human and experimental. Trans R Soc Med Hyg 70:374, 1976
6. Jones DB, Visvesvara GS, and Robinson NM: *Acanthamoeba polyphaga* keratitis and *Acanthamoeba* uveitis associated with fatal meningoencephalitis. Trans Ophthalmol Soc UK 95:221, 1975
7. Forster RK, Abbott RL, and Gelender H: Management of infectious endophthalmitis. Ophthalmol 87:313, 1980
8. Pavan-Langston D: Varicella-zoster ophthalmicus. Int Ophthalmol Clin 15:171, 1975
9. Meisler DM, Friedlaender MH, and Okumoto M: *Mycobacterium chelonei* keratitis. Am J Ophthalmol 94:398–401, 1982
10. Nozik RA: Personal communication
11. Brinser JH, and Burd EM: Principles of diagnostic ocular microbiology. In Tabbara KF, Hyndiuk RA (eds): Infections of the Eye, pp 73–92. Boston, Little Brown & Co, 1986
12. Friedlaender MH: Corticosteroid therapy of ocular inflammation. Int Ophthalmol Clin 23:175–82, 1983
13. Pfister R, and Paterson CA: Additional clinical and morphological observations on the favorable effect of ascorbate in experimental ocular alkali burns. Invest Ophthalmol Vis Sci 16:478, 1977

FIVE

Uveitic Glaucoma

Uveitic Glaucoma

Secondary uveitic glaucoma, one of the serious complications of intra-ocular inflammation,[1,2] occurs with various syndromes and may be difficult to manage. Most patients respond poorly to surgery. It is of primary importance to determine the severity of the inflammation and, if possible, the syndrome associated with it. Management includes treatment of the underlying inflammation and of the glaucoma itself. Various mechanisms produce secondary glaucoma, and it is important to identify them to institute the appropriate therapy.

Clinical Features

There is, in addition to the signs and symptoms of the underlying inflammation, an elevation of the intra-ocular pressure. If there is corneal disease or diffuse edema, the McKay-Marg tonometer or an air tonometer may be needed to measure accurately the intraocular pressure. Gonioscopy can determine whether or not there are synechiae or precipitates in the angle.

Pathology

The trabecular meshwork may be blocked with inflammatory cell debris or frank peripheral anterior synechiae. Iris bombé or rubeosis is also apparent in some cases.

TABLE 5-1. Uveitic Syndromes With Which Glaucoma May Be Associated

Posner-Schlossman syndrome (glaucomatocyclitic crisis)
Herpes simplex uveitis
Herpes zoster uveitis
Severe acute iridocyclitis
Rubella iridocyclitis
Nonspecific iridocyclitis
Fuchs' heterochromic iridocyclitis
Syphilitic uveitis
Iridocyclitis associated with ocular toxoplasmosis

Differential Diagnosis

Table 5-1 lists some of the major uveitic syndromes with which secondary glaucoma can be associated. Glaucoma may occur in any case of severe iridocyclitis, whatever the specific syndrome. Glaucoma secondary to peripheral anterior synechiae may develop late when the inflammation is no longer active.

The Posner-Schlossman syndrome (glaucomatocyclitic crisis) is characteristically intermittent with little evidence of inflammation.[3,4] Precipitates in the angle, however, may elevate the intra-ocular pressure considerably. Rubella, toxoplasmic-associated iridocyclitis herpes zoster, and herpes simplex are often accompanied by an elevation of pressure with relatively little anterior chamber inflammation. These diseases are accompanied by characteristic changes in the cornea and skin. Glaucoma occurs in up to 20% to 40% of Fuchs' heterochromic patients.[4]

Etiology

The two most common causes of secondary glaucoma in patients with uveitis are severe inflammation with blockage of the trabecular meshwork and peripheral anterior synechiae with secondary closure of the angle (Table 5-2). During the course of anterior uveitis, the trabecular meshwork may become completely or partially obstructed by inflammatory debris, mutton fat keratic precipitates, and particulate matter as well as inflammatory cells. Outflow facility may be further impaired by the increased viscosity of the aqueous humor, especially in an advanced and "plastic" iritis. Blood is often seen in Schlemm's canal in inflammatory processes, and indeed this is one of the hallmarks of Fuchs' heterochromic cyclitis. The meshwork may be overgrown by fibrous tissue or endothelium and Descemet's membrane. In addition, the inflammatory disease may involve the trabecular meshwork itself and further compromise its metabolism and function. The result is increased resistance to outflow of aqueous humor. However, inflammatory involvement of the ciliary body and the iris often alters the secretory pump and blood aqueous barrier in such a fashion that it results in a profound hyposecretion. Therefore, eyes with anterior uveitis are often in hypotony and the impaired outflow facility is not appreciated.

TABLE 5-2. Secondary Glaucoma: Causes, Incidence, and Treatment

Cause of Elevated Intra-ocular Pressure	Incidence	Topical and Systemic Treatment
Blockage of trabecula with debris	Common	Therapy for inflammation
Peripheral anterior synechiae	Common	Carbonic anhydrase inhibitors, timolol, epinephrine
Iris bombé	Rare	Iridectomy
Trabeculitis (Posner-Schlossman syndrome)	Rare	Carbonic anhydrase inhibitors, timolol, epinephrine, standard treatment for inflammation
Rubeosis iridis	Rare	Carbonic anhydrase inhibitors, timolol, epinephrine, cyclocryotherapy
Hypersecretion	Extremely rare	Carbonic anhydrase inhibitors, timolol, epinephrine
Sclerosis of the trabecular meshwork	Not known	Carbonic anhydrase inhibitors, timolol, epinephrine
Corticosteroid-induced	3%–10%	Discontinue corticosteroids

The administration of steroids or the spontaneous cessation of the inflammatory process may restore secretion, while the outflow facility may still be impaired. This results in a pressure elevation. In a chronic anterior uveitis, the damage to the trabecular meshwork may be more permanent but still not visible gonioscopically. In herpes zoster opthalmicus with secondary uveitis, for example, as many as 25% of the affected eyes are found to have elevations of the intra-ocular pressure. Often unrecognized, this becomes an exceptionally difficult clinical dilemma, especially when one wants to diminish steroid dependence in herpetic patients in whom one suspects that the elevation may be due to trabecular damage as well as to an accommodation to the steroid itself.

The treatment of secondary glaucoma, due to active anterior uveitis, is directed at the inflammatory process itself. Efforts must be made to dilate the pupil with midriatics and cycloplegics and to decrease inflammatory reaction to such a degree that damage, scarring, and visual loss are minimized at best. Corticosteroids are particularly useful for this purpose. Their prolonged use may prove necessary, and one must then try to differentiate possible elevations of intraocular pressure caused by the steroids rather than by the original disease process. In unilateral conditions, a corticosteroid provocative test in the normal eye may permit such a differentiation and pinpoint whether the eye is responding to the steroid with pressure elevation. In some of the more difficult situations, intra-ocular pressure alternates between disease cause and steroid-induced elevation. In all inflammatory processes, the clinician hopes that the outflow mechanism will ultimately restore itself to normal. As long as the outflow facility is impaired, pressure should be maintained within normal limits by the addition of topical β-blocking agents, epinephrine, systemic carbonic anhydrase inhibitors, and even resorting to osmotic agents. When the inflammatory process is no longer active, miotics may prove helpful.

Treatment

Special consideration should be given to the management of acute intra-ocular inflammation with elevated intra-ocular pressure. If it is certain that corticosteroids are not the cause of the elevated pressure, the following regimen is suggested:

1. A strong topical corticosteroid is instilled every hour during the day and every 2 hours during the night.
2. Acetazolamide, 250 mg every 8 hours, or 500 mg sequel every 12 hours, is prescribed.
3. Epinephrine 1% solution every 12 hours and/or timolol maleate 0.5% solution every 12 hours is given.
4. Cycloplegics are administered three or four times per day.
5. Systemic prednisone, 60 mg, is given every morning; if inflammation is severe, a sub-Tenon's capsule injection of moderately long-acting corticosteroid is used.

Miotics usually are contraindicated in acute inflammatory glaucoma. Because epinephrine occasionally causes headaches and discomfort, timolol is rapidly becoming the drug of choice for nonspecific inflammatory glaucoma. On the other hand, most ocular inflammations, with acute secondary glaucoma due to blockage of the angle by inflammatory cells, improve after just a few days of corticosteroid therapy.

Corticosteroid-induced glaucoma is a major differential diagnostic problem when it complicates intra-ocular inflammation. Usually the glaucoma does not develop until at least 4 to 6 weeks after the corticosteroid therapy is begun. If the inflammation responds well to the corticosteroid, sub-Tenon's capsule and subconjunctival depot preparations should be avoided. Frequently the clinician must balance the benefit conferred by the corticosteroid against the limited ability of the eye to tolerate elevations of pressure. If the glaucoma cannot be controlled, it may be necessary to remove surgically a previously injected depot preparation. A patient with corticosteroid-induced glaucoma often requires maximum medical therapy for both the glaucoma and the inflammation, and the clinician must prescribe other anti-inflammatory drugs.

Surgical Procedures in Secondary Glaucoma and Inflammatory Glaucoma

The preferred procedure for iris bombé is surgical iridectomy, since transfixation of the iris or laser iridotomy is often followed by rapid occlusion of the small openings. Iridotomy should be performed under general anesthesia or, if the eye is not too inflamed, local anesthesia. At the same time, a sub-Tenon's capsule injection of corticosteroids may be given.

The results of filtering surgery often are not good. For this surgery, the eye should be as uninflamed as possible. While laser trabeculoplasty may be tried (if the angle is open), results have not been encouraging[5,6] and surgical intervention is usually required later. Standard trabeculectomy or other filtering procedures such as modified goniotomy, thermal sclerostomy, and posterior lip sclerotomy have afforded limited success.[7,8,9] A standard filtering procedure (thermal sclerostomy preferred), however, has a greater chance of success if the eye has been quiet for several months than when the eye has been quiet for a shorter time. Krupin-Denver or Molteno valves may be important as well.[10,11] A laser iridotomy may be elected to "break" an attack until a standard surgery can be performed.

If both filtering surgery and maximal medical therapy have failed, cyclocryotherapy is recommended. Unfortunately, this procedure causes significant inflammation and a definite risk of phthisis bulbi. Thus it is a procedure of last resort.

Cyclocryotherapy can be performed in a number of ways. The glaucoma cryoprobe can be used under local anesthesia. The inferior 180 degrees of the eye is treated with two rows of "freeze" for 1 minute at −80°C in three spots per quadrant. The first row begins about 2 mm to 3 mm behind the limbus, with the "ice ball" extending partially onto the cornea. The second row is placed immediately behind the first. By freezing two separate rows, the need to freeze and then refreeze is eliminated. The eye is patched after the instillation of a combined corticosteroid and antibiotic together with a cycloplegic. Because patients experience significant pain in the postoperative period, an effective analgesic is important.

Synechiae

Synechiae, leading to iris bombé and pupillary block in the phakic and pseudophakic patient, may be treated with a YAG laser with extreme caution. Phakic patients, of course, run the risk of cataract development and lens-induced uveitis if the anterior lens capsule suffers inadvertent microscopic rupture. This can be avoided if the focus is decentered (0.1 to 0.3 mm), and the absolute area between synechiae and the iris ruff is carefully lased (Fig. 5-1, 5-2). If one lyses the synechiae from the iris collarette surface, even though its distal remnant still adheres to the anterior lens capsule, often they will release or can be "unzipped." The adhesion will open, however, and there is instantaneous release of the bombé. Because of the release (a "mini-shower") of pigment, it is advisable to treat the patient postoperatively with steroid drops as well as to keep the pupil "moving" with 2.5% neo-synephrine for the ensuing few days. If the underlying iridocyclitis is intercurrent, new synechiae formation will occur rapidly. Should

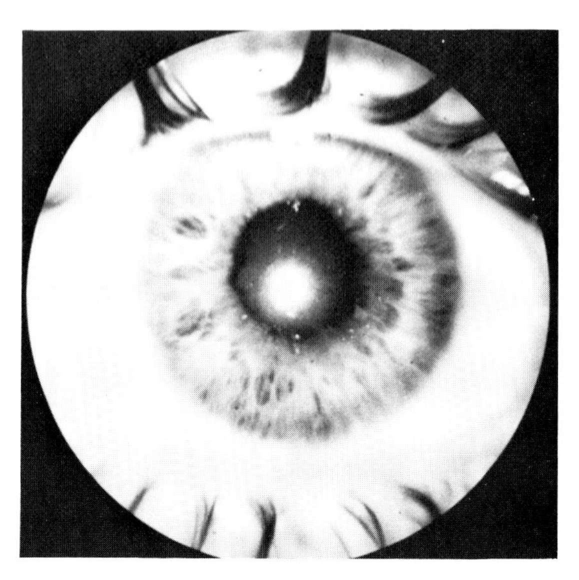

Figure 5-1. A 24-year-old phakic male patient with Reiter's disease, acute iritis, and iris bombé. The heavy synechiae at the 9:00 to 12:00 position were broken using a YAG laser, being careful to place the spots on the iris ruff, forward of the anterior lens capsule.

this situation occur, every attempt should be made to suppress the intraocular inflammation.

Specific Uveitic Glaucoma Syndromes

Fuchs' Heterochromic Cyclitis

Heterochromic cyclitis is one type of usually mild uveitis that often retains an open angle but demonstrates keratic precipitates. Insidious pressure rises are found in some 20% of hypochromic eyes. Twig-like and sausage-like neovascularizations of the iris periphery and trabecular meshwork are often seen in this condition. In former times, paracentesis of the anterior chamber, to provoke bleeding from these aberrant vessels, was often considered a diagnostic test for Fuchs' heterochromic cyclitis. Thus, hyphema may be a frequent complication of minor trauma to these eyes. Cataracts occur in 85% of eyes with heterochromic cyclitis. A lens extraction is well tolerated in spite of recurrent hyphema. Because this may be a mild type of uveitis, the future findings may prove these cases able to tolerate intra-ocular lens implantation fairly well (Fig. 5-3). Therapy for iridocyclitis is relatively ineffective in Fuchs' heterochromic cyclitis. Most important

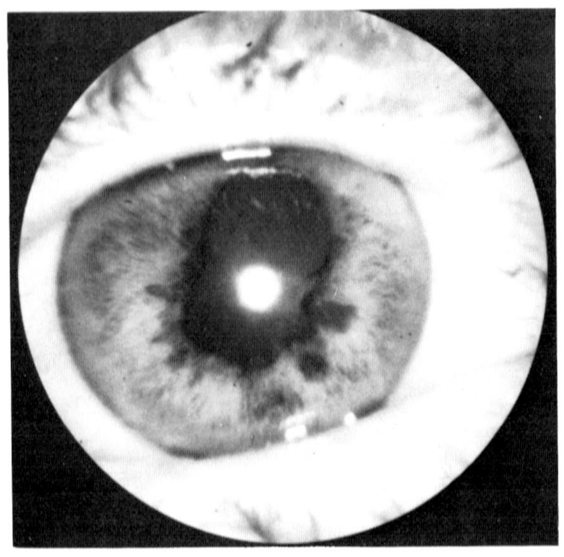

Figure 5-2. A 36-year-old phakic female patient with posterior synechiae for 360-degree and pupil-block glaucoma. The heavy synechiae at the 3:30 to 6:00 position were released at the iris ruff without harm to the anterior lens capsule.

in differential diagnosis are those instances in heterochromia with pressure elevation on the more pigmented side. This occurs in diffuse iris melanoma as well and in hemosiderosis or siderosis bulbae. An ultimate glaucoma, which is especially unamenable to medical or surgical treatment, often seems to become fixed in these eyes. One may have to result to surgical trabeculectomy as an ultimate procedure for the deep-seated and difficult-to-manage glaucoma that occurs in some 75%–80% of patients with heterochromic cyclitis after about 10 years of recurrent inflammatory glaucoma (Fig. 5-4).

Glaucomatocyclitic Crisis

Posner-Schlossmann syndrome is a distinct entity falling into the category of secondary open angle glaucoma with uveitis. It is characterized by minimal inflammatory signs and symptoms, and synechiae are extremely rare. The inflammatory disease may be confined entirely to the trabecular meshwork as a "trabeculitis." The process is usually unilateral with recurrent involvement of the same eye. Occasional bilateral cases are seen with both eyes involved at the same time or on different occasions.

Bilaterality or more impressive inflammatory signs should suggest careful re-examination of the fundus, particularly the far periphery, for chorioretinitis and inflammatory lesions since these can closely resemble a glaucomatocyclitic

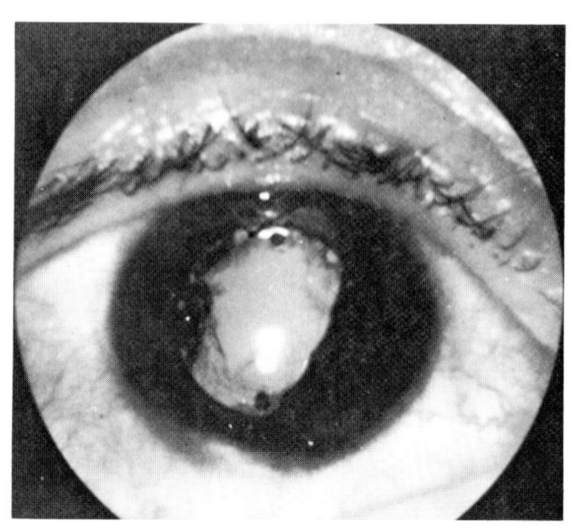

Figure 5-3. A 62-year-old patient with postoperative uveitis, with pupil block glaucoma, whose synchiae from the 2:00 to 6:00 position were lysed free from the posterior chamber lens, re-establishing a normal pressure, without laser "nicks" on the I.O.L.

crisis picture in the anterior chamber. In contrast to the small pupil of anterior uveitis, eyes with glaucomatocyclitic crisis usually have a dilated pupil. The patients have remarkably few symptoms relative to the height of the intra-ocular pressure. Their first complaint may be blurring of vision due to a transient corneal edema, which may even disappear overnight. During attacks of pressure elevation, which rarely last more than two weeks, the angles remain open, and any change in the usual field would be distinctly unusual. During an attack, usually immediately following pressure normalization, cells and flare will be seen in the anterior chamber and keratic precipitates (KP) may often appear—usually as a few, discrete, nongranulomatous KP. During the attack, the outflow facility is markedly depressed but it usually returns to normal between episodes. There is rarely ever permanent alteration in outflow facility. Surgery is almost always contraindicated in glaucomatocyclitic crisis. It is best treated with mild mydriatics, topical steroids, topical β-blockers, epinephrine, and systemic carbonic anhydrase inhibitors.

Lens-Induced Glaucomas

The lens may play an important role in many of the secondary inflammatory glaucomas. Traumatic or spontaneous subluxation of the lens can result in glaucoma with angle closure due to pupil block with either the vitreous gel or the lens itself. In many instances of lens subluxation, the outflow facility is decreased in both eyes without angle closure. However traumatic, lens subluxation may have

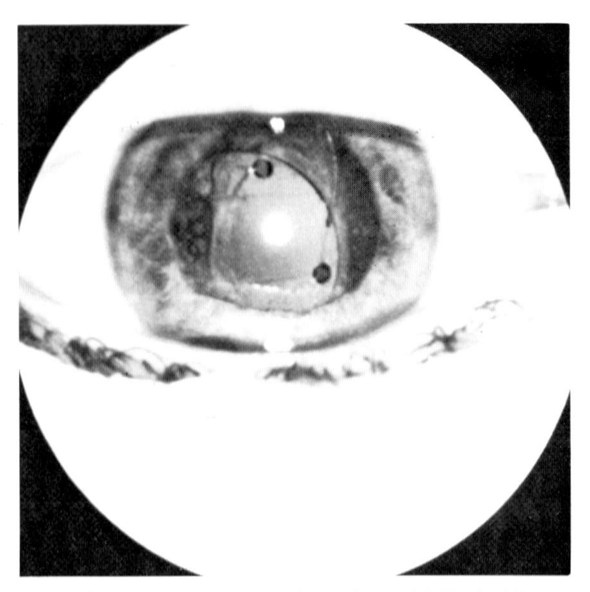

Figure 5-4. A 57-year-old male patient with Fuchs' heterochromic cyclitis after extracapsular cataract extraction and posterior chamber lens placement. In the dilated position one can note a slightly decentered I.O.L., but a central clear capsulotomy. This particular category of patient (Fuchs' heterochromic cyclitis) does well with posterior chamber intraocular lens placement, while it is contraindicated in most other categories of uveitis/glaucoma.

synechiae associated with it, either in the angle or in the pupillary margin, and vitreous may also play a role in blocking the angle. Some of these lens subluxations are explained as congenital anomalies of the angle (e.g., in Marfan's syndrome) and are not necessarily a consequence of lens dislocation itself. Other lens dislocations may be associated with an inflammatory disease such as syphilis and secondary glaucoma. In some lens dislocations, as in homocystenuria, open-angle glaucoma has not been described but anterior dislocation with acute pressure elevations has been seen. Many eyes, particularly those with traumatic posterior subluxation of the lens, have impaired outflow facility and have abnormally deep anterior chambers and recessed angles. The mechanism by which the outflow facility is impaired in these instances is not clear. It may be related to the trauma rather than to the dislocated lens itself. Removal of the lens is indicated only if vision is impaired by the lens or if a phakolytic inflammation ensues, whereby a rent in the lens capsule itself leaks antigenic protein which sets up an unremitting inflammatory state. This inflammatory state usually is not amenable to medical management with corticosteroids. Cryostatic methods have most often proved useful in removing such a dislocated lens. This may be one of the only indications left in ophthalmology today for which cryoprobe extraction of a lens, on an intracapsular basis, is the treatment of choice. Removal of the lens may not reverse the glaucomatous process, and further medical or surgical treatment may be necessary to lessen the pressure elevation and ameliorate the inflammatory state that coexists with it.

Phacolytic Glaucoma

In phacolytic glaucoma, the trabecular meshwork is blocked by macrophages containing lens material. In these eyes the anterior chambers are deep, the angles are open, the cataract is often hypermature and may be white with distinct color changes giving it the appearance of a bag of fluid rather than a proteinaceous lens. The patient may possess only faulty light projection. Early in the disease process, the inflammatory reaction is minimal, with a few clumps of macrophages on the back of the cornea and an impaired outflow facility. As the disease progresses, however, there is a marked elevation of intra-ocular pressure—often with corneal edema, congestion, and pain. In many cases, the phacolytic glaucoma is believed to result from leakage of lens material through a faulty lens capsule or rent in its front surface and into the anterior chamber. In some instances there may be a frank rupture of the capsule. Often, however, this disease progresses so rapidly by the leeching of antigenic protein into the anterior chamber that, by the time one sees the patient, there is such a steamy cornea that adequate visualization of structures in the anterior chamber is no longer possible. Macrophages filled with lens material are found not only in the trabecular meshwork, but also on the surface of the iris and on the back of the cornea. It has recently been stated that 25% or more of eyes with phacolytic glaucoma coming to histopathologic examination have recessed angles. The differential diagnosis of phacolytic glaucoma must include (1) a swollen cataractous lens that itself has induced-angle closure, but which may be easily recognized by gonioscopy and (2) a lens-induced uveitis with glaucoma, in which the glaucoma is related to the inflammatory reaction or its sequelae.

The treatment of a phacolytic glaucoma should consist of prompt measures to lower the intra-ocular pressure. This is usually done with the instillation of a beta blocker such as timolol, epinephrine, Propine, and carbonic anhydrase inhibitors. Concomitant instillation of corticosteroids to decrease the inflammatory component is usually necessary. Prompt extraction of the lens after the intra-ocular pressure is reduced is the actual treatment of the disease process. The removal of the lens often results in normalization of outflow facility and intra-ocular pressure, and frequently no further treatment is required. Even in a patient with bare light perception and projection preoperatively, surprisingly good vision may be obtained after this crisis of intra-ocular pressure elevation usually with an intense inflammatory component.

Lens-Induced Uveitis

Lens-induced uveitis results from reactions to lens material either through the intact capsule or after spontaneous rupture or extracapsular extraction of a mature cataract. The process is characterized by marked excitation of lymphocytes and plasma cells, invasion of the lens by leukocytes, much reaction in the anterior chamber, and conglomerate precipitates on the back of the cornea which are large, greasy, and "mutton fat" in character. The eyes are often soft at the time of the acute reaction, but after the development of synechiae, fibrous membranes, and scarring, and intense glaucoma may ensue. Cataract extraction or removal of cortical material with a vitrectomy instrument is curative in these cases of uveitis and results in the avoidance or the amelioration of the glaucomatous process itself.

Traumatic Glaucoma

Traumatic penetrating injuries from a variety of sharp or toxic objects such as toys, glass, wire, knives, and scissors may result in an inflammatory glaucoma. The type of glaucoma resulting from such an injury usually is dependent upon the position or extent of the injury, the skill of the surgeon in repairing damage, and the post-traumatic inflammatory reaction of the eye. The initial repair of the injury is often of greater importance in maintaining a useful eye than any of the subsequent operations to counteract the secondary inflammatory glaucoma. This is usually true also in instances of siderosis that may cause an ongoing inflammatory reaction in the eye.

The blow of a blunt object to the eye may result in a sudden increase in intra-ocular pressure and a variety of injuries to the intra-ocular contents. In the anterior segment, the iris may be suddenly forced against the lens by pressure of the aqueous humor and by stretching of the posterior sclera. The valve-like action of the iris prevents aqueous humor from running back through the pupil, and the pressure may cause a blowout of the peripheral iris termed an *iridodialysis.* This anatomic flattening of the pupil on the side of the tear and displacement of the pupil away from that area is an important sign. Diathermy or argon laser treatment may be needed at a later date to stop recurrent bleeding from such an iris tear. There may also be a telltale tear of the pupil or of the sphincter, but these usually bleed less frequently.

A more frequent and potentially more serious problem is produced if the iris tear occurs all the way back into the ciliary body, ripping into that structure. This is the usual source of severe recurrent hemorrhages into the anterior chamber and vitreous gel that so often lead to loss of an eye. More often tears into the ciliary body result with the gonioscopic picture of a recessed angle. Usually within 1 to 2 hours after a severe blunt trauma, the intra-ocular pressure may increase markedly. This results from the red cells or from the erythrocytes obstructing the trabecular meshwork or even from acute edematous contusion of the outflow channels themselves. The inflammatory glaucoma that results from such a blunt injury often subsides in 24 to 72 hours and is usually followed, interestingly, by a period of marked hypotony. The patient, however, may require frequent doses of hyperosmotic agents to lower the pressure during the acute phase and until the hypotony occurs. In the few eyes that demonstrate angle recession, there is usually a secondary rise in intra-ocular pressure which occurs late. It can begin 1 to 2 months after injury and, if controlled medically, may spontaneously subside within a year or two and disappear completely, requiring no further medication or treatment. In some instances, however, particularly when the angle recession is extensive, there may be the late development of open-angle glaucoma. This can occur even 5 to 10 years after injury. It is usually readily differentiated from primary glaucoma by the gonioscopic appearance of the angle and its unilaterality. Gonioscopically, the most important characteristic sign is a widening of the distance from the scleral spur to the iris root, resulting in a broadened ciliary band in the area of the recession. A localized deepening of the anterior chamber is frequent, and remnants of torn iris tissue and scattered pigmentary change may be seen along the margins of the tear. Segmental disruption of the iris processes is a helpful sign when present. Occasionally the signs are quite subtle and only gonioscopic comparison, back and forth, between the two eyes, demonstrates the abnormality.

Although angle recession is common after traumatic hyphema, the vast majority of eyes with recessed angles fail to actually develop glaucoma or any evidence of outflow impairment. It is apparent that a recessed angle is a symbol of injury to the eye and a rough measure of the severity of the injury, but it is not always synonymous with glaucoma nor is the recession necessarily causative in the development of pressure elevation. The recessed angle, the intra-ocular pressure elevation, and lens dislocation, when present, are merely all consequences of trauma. It is important to look specifically for recessed angles in all unilaterally glaucomatous eyes and particularly in those with a history of blunt trauma. A blowout into the subchoroidal space can occur producing a cyclodialysis. This rarely happens and usually leads to severe hypotony and cataract formation and not necessarily to a glaucomatous crisis.

Hemorrhagic Glaucoma

Spontaneous or traumatic hemorrhages into the anterior chamber, particularly if recurrent, can be an important cause of secondary glaucoma in the inflammatory state. After many types of trauma or inflammation, there is often a rise of intra-ocular pressure for a short period of time. This is usually followed by more prolonged hypotony, especially in eyes with chronic uveitis. If trauma has resulted in sufficient hemorrhage into the anterior chamber to block the outflow channels, a marked rise in intra-ocular pressure may ensue when secretion recovers at the ciliary body. If this is allowed to persist, bloodstaining of the cornea as well as severe damage to the optic nerve may occur. Even in instances in which hemorrhage into the anterior chamber is less profound, breakdown products of the blood itself, perhaps even iron, may result in permanent damage to the outflow channels with a resulting hemosiderosis. The impaired outflow facility may present a picture of chronic, unilateral open-angle glaucoma that is difficult to distinguish clinically or histologically from primary glaucoma. The finding of traumatic recession of the angle is an important differential sign.

The treatment of an anterior chamber hemorrhage after trauma or uveitis should consist of patching the eye or considering sedentary bed rest for the patient, with sufficient sedation to make this regimen tolerable to a child as well as to an adult. Rarely need the patient be hospitalized for observation. Usually no drops are used unless signs of severe iritis are present, in which case mild mydriatics are then indicated. If there has been no hemorrhage after 5 days, the regimen can be discontinued. The recurrence of hemorrhage is more common on the second to fourth day and is accompanied by an increased intra-ocular pressure. This is best treated with systemic carbonic anhydrase inhibitors and with topical epinephrine drops. If hemorrhage and increased pressure cannot be controlled, a steamy cornea ensues or if bloodstaining has started to occur, then acute elevations of intra-ocular pressure may require oral glycerol or even intravenous urea of mannitol. A change in the color of the blood in the anterior chamber, from bright red to black, usually indicates breakdown of the hemoglobin molecules. This is often the forerunner of bloodstaining of the cornea that can persist for months to years. If the intra-ocular pressure cannot be controlled by medical means or if the anterior chamber remains completely filled with blood, the blood should be washed out to avoid possible bloodstaining. Preoperative hyperosmotic therapy usually simplifies the operation and makes it safer. Occasionally such lowering of intraocular pressure hastens the blood reabsorption and further surgery is avoided. Procrastination may result in more trabecular damage, with anterior synechiae formation and a chronic glaucoma that is very difficult to manage, as well as bloodstaining of the cornea and optic nerve cupping.

The use of a 20-gauge needle on a syringe containing a highly purified fibrinolysin or kinase (urokinase) of human origin will facilitate the lysis and washing out of clots. This may be accomplished by general irrigation back and forth into the syringe. This is usually better facilitated with the use of an irrigating, aspirating instrument, a usual I-A type instrument or one of the vitrectomy instruments. After the anterior chamber is cleared of blood, an air bubble is introduced, and it may become a very effective tamponade. If this procedure fails to remove the blood, it is safest to turn down a conjunctival flap, place a McLean suture, and enter the anterior chamber through an *ab-externo* incision. Blood should be washed out through a small incision if possible. Often the blood can be removed only by extending the incision and pulling out the clotted material with forceps or "eating" it out with a vitrectomy instrument. In some cases a small circle of diathermic coagulation, 3 mm back from the limbus at the suspected site of the bleeding, may be helpful in preventing a recurring hemorrhage postoperatively.

In eyes that have suffered sufficient trabecular damage or have formed sufficient anterior synechiae, chronic glaucoma will develop. These eyes should be treated like other chronic secondary glaucomas. Preference should be given to medical therapy using strong myotics and carbonic anhydrase inhibitors. Any persistence or recurrence of iridocyclitis should be treated with corticosteroids and mydriatics. The patient should be warned of the danger of a chronic glaucoma occurring from an initial injury or from uveitic damage to the structures at once or even years after.

Intra-ocular Foreign Bodies

Intra-ocular foreign bodies are dealt with in Chapter 11. There are certain concepts, however, which are germane to a discussion of glaucoma in these inflammatory situations. Damage to the eye from an intra-ocular foreign body may not be confined to the lens, vitreous, and retina but may also involve the trabecular meshwork. Siderosis from an iron foreign body not only decreases outflow facility, but produces alterations in the structure of the trabecular meshwork itself that closely resemble primary open-angle glaucoma. The resulting open-angle glaucoma is usually difficult, if not impossible, to control. Therapy in these cases consists in the immediate removal of the foreign body, when known to be of iron-containing material, before there is damage to the outflow channels. When glaucoma already exists, the treatment should be the same as for any other open-angle glaucoma.

References

1. Intraocular Inflammation, Uveitis, and Ocular Tumors. Ophthalmology Basic and Clinical Science Course (Section 3). San Francisco, American Academy of Ophthalmology, 1981–1982
2. Smith RE, Nozik RM: Uveitis: A Clinical Approach to Diagnosis and Management. Baltimore, Williams & Wilkins, 1983
3. DeRoetth A Jr: Glaucomatocyclitic crisis. Am J Ophthalmol 69:370, 1970
4. Kass MA, Becker B, Kolker AE: Glaucomatocyclitic crisis and primary open-angle glaucoma. Am J Ophthalmol 75:668, 1973
5. Lieberman MF, Hoskins HD, Hetherington J: Laser trabeculoplasty and the glaucomas. Ophthalmology 90:790, 1983
6. Robin AL, Pollack IP: Argon laser trabeculoplasty in secondary forms of open-angle glaucoma. Arch Ophthalmol 3:382, 1983
7. Singh D, Singh M: Pretrabecular filtration for secondary glaucoma. Trans Ophthalmol Soc UK 98:96, 1978
8. Herschler J, Davis EB: Modified goniotomy for inflammatory glaucoma: Histologic evidence for the mechanism of pressure reduction. Arch Ophthalmol 98:684, 1980
9. Sugar HS: Limbal trephination: A twenty-year follow-up. Int Ophthalmol Clin 21:29, 1981
10. Molteno ACB: A new implant for glaucoma: Clinical trial. Br J Ophthalmol 53:606, 1969
11. Krupin T, Rodos SM et al: Valve implants in filtering surgery. Am J Ophthalmol 81:232, 1976

SIX

Cataract Extraction in Patients With Uveitis

Cataract extraction poses significant risks for patients with uveitis.[1] The outcome of such surgery often depends upon the particular uveitis syndrome.

The less inflamed the eye at the time of surgery, the better the prognosis and the less the chance of severe postoperative complications. Treating inflamed eyes with high doses of corticosteroids (systemically, topically, or by sub-Tenon's capsule injection) for a few days or a week before surgery is recommended. If posterior inflammation threatens the outcome, such as in recurrent retinal vasculitis, it is wise to defer surgery until the inflammation subsides, either naturally or with medication.

In many uveitis syndromes, cataract may be caused by the inflammation itself, which produces significant lens opacity, or by the chronic use of corticosteroids, which are cataractogenic.

The indications for cataract extraction in patients with ocular inflammation are visual disability, "maturity" of the cataract, and lens-induced inflammation. If the eye has been quiet without medications and there has been no active inflammation for at least several months, a routine lens extraction usually can be performed without significant risk. But when inflammation (even low-grade) is present, special precautions and surgical techniques are necessary.

If the cataract is mature and there is significant capsular involvement or liquefaction of cortical material, extraction is advisable to prevent lens-induced disorders from being superimposed on an underlying inflammatory process.

The only urgent indication for cataract surgery is a uveitis that appears to have been caused by the lens material itself. Phacoanaphylaxis, phacolytic glaucoma with cataract, and "phacotoxic" reactions caused by residual lens material after extracapsular lens extractions indicate that the lens or lens material should be removed to eliminate the cause of the active inflammation. If all of the lens material is not removed, the inflammation may persist indefinitely.

Specific Uveitic Syndromes

Juvenile Rheumatoid Arthritis and Iridocyclitis

Earlier results of extracapsular cataract extraction in patients with juvenile rheumatoid arthritis were not encouraging as the sequelae were frequent vitreous loss and incarcerations in the cataract wound, development of cyclitic membranes, and subsequent ciliary body detachment with eventual phthisis. One report of 15 cases, in which standard extracapsular techniques were used (e.g., aspiration), cited 11 patients with no light perception by the end of 5 years.[2] A more encouraging report came from the Proctor Foundation in San Francisco: vision of 20/200 was achieved in 60% of patients.[3] With lensectomy-vitrectomy surgery, capsule remnants, cyclitic membranes, and calcified particles can be removed more completely, thus lessening significantly the possible outcome of ciliary body detachment and phthisis.

If patients with juvenile rheumatoid arthritis have progressive cataract and extraction of the lens is indicated, combined lensectomy and subtotal vitrectomy performed through the limbus or pars plana is recommended (Figs. 6-1, 6-2).

Fuchs' Heterochromic Iridocyclitis

Although earlier reports indicated that bleeding from abnormal angle vessels was a serious complication after cataract extraction in patients with Fuchs' heterochromic cyclitis,[4,5] this was not proved to be a consistent complication in any of 29 cases reviewed by Smith and O'Connor.[6] Results from the Mayo Clinic have suggested a slight increase in complications following routine cataract extraction in Fuchs' patients.[7] In general, however, any standard procedure for cataract surgery usually can be used without significant risk of intra-operative or postoperative complications. Transient postoperative hyphemas may occur but seldom create a long-term problem. Since Fuchs' cyclitis is generally unilateral, the usual indications for this type of cataract extraction apply. The patient's vision may not return to 20/20, however, because the disease can cause visually impairing vitreous opacities.

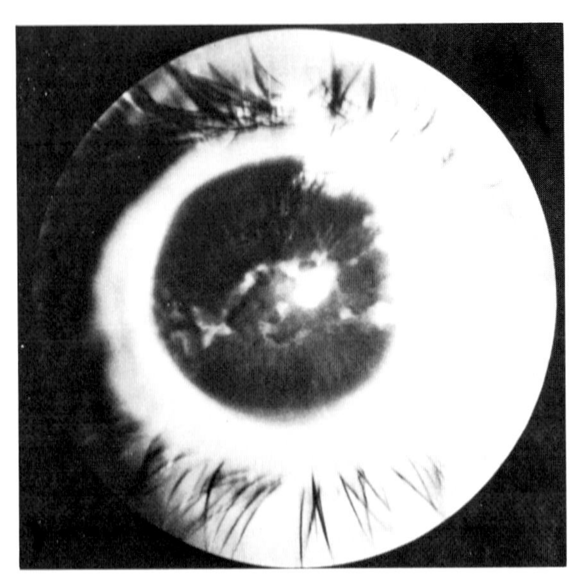

Figure 6-1. A 27-year-old white woman with phthisical eye, band keratopathy, secluded fibrosed pupil, and dense cataract (demonstrated by ultrasonography) due to juvenile rheumatoid arthritis.

Pars Planitis (Chronic Cyclitis, Peripheral Uveitis, Intermediate Uveitis)

Pars planitis is a chronic, bilateral uveitis characterized by persistent vitreous cells, opacities, and low-grade anterior chamber inflammation that may last for several years. Lens opacities develop in a significant number of cases (42%), but little information is available concerning the prognosis for cataract surgery. Smith and co-workers[8] described intracapsular and extracapsular lens extractions in 21 eyes with chronic cyclitis. Of these, 13 had vision of better than 20/40 several years after the surgery. Complications were not significantly higher than in patients in whom there was no inflammation, and no cases of phthisis or prolonged reactivation of inflammation were noted. Diamond and Kaplan[9,10] reported several cases of combined lensectomy-vitrectomy in pars planitis patients with no significant complications.

Pars planitis does not seem to increase the risk of complications in routine intracapsular or extracapsular cataract surgery. However, postoperative vision is limited by the complications of the disease itself: cystoid macular edema and vitreous opacities. Although routine cataract extraction can be performed safely, combined lensectomy-vitrectomy may be preferred for such patients, because vitreous opacities are a significant problem postoperatively. Diamond and Kaplan[9,10] have suggested removing the vitreous to lessen cystoid macular edema. More data on the effectiveness of this approach are needed.

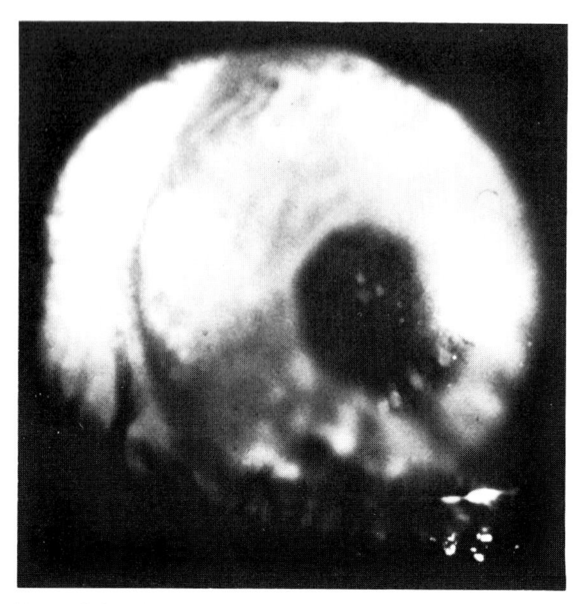

Figure 6-2. After removal of band keratopathy and lensectomy/vitrectomy, the vision improved from light perception to 20/80, with a rise in intraocular pressure from 2 mm Hg to 8 mm Hg. The eye is micro-ophthalmic.

Lens-Induced Uveitis (Phacoanaphylactic Endophthalmitis, Phacolytic Glaucoma, Phacotoxic Uveitis)

Phacoanaphylactic endophthalmitis is a sterile granulomatous inflammatory response to lens material. It is secondary to autosensitization to the patient's own lens protein. It typically occurs after traumatic or surgical rupture of the lens capsule with escape of cortical material. The capsular rupture apparently exposes the normally sequestered lens substance to the body's immune system, the capsule having previously formed a protective barrier.

In rare instances, an otherwise successful intra-ocular lens (IOL) implantation after an extracapsular cataract extraction (ECCE) can be complicated by a noninfectious inflammatory process that is refractory to treatment, including removal of the IOL. It is important that the implant surgeon be aware that the inflammatory reaction may not be a result of the IOL itself, but rather a hypersensitivity reaction to the patient's own lens protein. This protein, derived from residual lens material following ECCE, may cause a transient phacotoxic response that usually subsides rapidly, or it may induce a true phacoanaphylactic reaction.[12]

With the present and ever-increasing transition from intracapsular cataract extraction (ICCE) to ECCE, it might be expected that phacoanaphylaxis may now occur again with higher frequency. Yet, this disorder is still relatively rare, probably due to marked improvement in ECCE techniques. However, this disease is easily overlooked and its diagnosis may be difficult. Therefore, the incidence is clearly higher than indicated by published reports.

The onset of a phacoanaphylactic reaction typically occurs between 1 and 14 days after traumatic or surgical capsular disruption. However, extremes have been reported in which the reaction occurred as early as several hours, or as late as several months, following capsular rupture. Brinkman and Broekhuyse (cited by Apple et al[18]) feel that the clinical response of a rapid phacoanaphylaxis represents a secondary immune response to leaking lenticular antigens following capsular rupture in a patient who is already immunologically primed with sensitized lymphocytes. An occasional associated sympathetic response in the fellow eye has been documented.[12]

Phacoanaphylactic endophthalmitis is characterized histologically by a zonal granulomatous inflammatory reaction about the lens or lens remnants.[19-21] There is a central polymorphonuclear reaction that is surrounded by concentric layers of various inflammatory cells, including epithelioid and giant cells. The adjacent iris and ciliary body typically show an infiltration of plasma cells and lymphocytes. The entire mass may become encased in granulation tissue. Foamy macrophages have been seen in eyes with phacoanaphylactic uveitis.[22] They may be similar to the foamy macrophages classically associated with phacolytic glaucoma.

The implant surgeon should be aware of the possibility of post-ECCE phacoanaphylactic uveitis in cases where the etiology of postoperative inflammation is obscure, especially if the fellow eye has already been operated with ECCE. Removal of the IOL will *not* be curative. In rare cases, the inflammatory process will resolve with aggressive corticosteroid therapy. Otherwise, the only effective treatment is complete removal of residual lens cortical material and thorough cleansing of the anterior segment. An ECCE should not be performed on the opposite eye, and this eye should be carefully followed to rule out a possible sympathizing response.

If unrecognized and thus untreated, phacoanaphylactic endophthalmitis may lead to any of the sequelae of chronic inflammation, including phthisis bulbi.

Once the diagnosis of lens-induced uveitis is established, the lens should be extracted and the residual lens material removed as soon as possible.[11,14] In the case of phacoanaphylactic endophthalmitis, careful removal of all lens material also is important. Depending on the patient, an intracapsular extraction may be possible, but more often is not. A careful and complete extracapsular extraction by means of microsurgical techniques is the alternative.

Although the lens is usually intact in patients with phacolytic glaucoma, it is often quite fragile, and attempts at intracapsular surgery may rupture the capsule. If this occurs, it is necessary to convert the procedure to an extracapsular one and to remove all lens material. Before surgery in such patients, high doses of corticosteroids (given systemically, subconjunctivally, and topically) and osmotic agents may be needed to control the intra-ocular pressure.

The most important aspects in the management of such patients are the correct diagnosis, control of the intra-ocular pressure and inflammation, and the removal of all lens material, preferably by an intracapsular procedure. These cases are considered semi-emergencies and the patient should be operated on as soon as possible.

Intra-ocular Lens-Induced Uveitis

Intra-ocular inflammation may result as a consequence of a misplaced or displaced intra-ocular lens whose structure is causing disruption of iris, pigment, or stroma. Older modeled implants, those with titanium clips or ill-fitting Choyce-style lenses whose haptics "jammed" into the angle and trabecular meshwork, were examples of uveitis-inducing lenses.[23,24] Such was the etiology of "UGH" syndrome: a smoldering intractable uveitis due to corrosion of intra-ocular tissue made manifest by uveitis, glaucoma, and hyphema necessitating removal of the offending implant. The eponym "UGH" for this complication of the early generation intra-ocular lenses was first coined by Ellingson.[24] He noted also that some of the Choyce-style anterior chamber lenses had warped foot plates that, in addition to causing the corrosion problem, produced a rocking motion of the lens. This induced a mechanical irritation at the root of the iris and on adjacent structures of the anterior chamber,[23,24] which resulted in uveitis, recurrent hyphema, and glaucoma. This combination of signs gave rise to the UGH eponym: uveitis, glaucoma, hyphema. This condition usually subsided following removal of the implant. As Figure 6-1 shows, a considerable anterior segment inflammation is found in this patient with UGH syndrome whose eye quieted almost immediately after removal of the lens; however, persistent cystoid macular edema and crenated keratic precipitates remained for 6 months after lens removal, but then vision returned to normal.

Keates and Ehrlich[25] described 12 intra-ocular lenses removed due to UGH syndrome and documented upon removal of these lenses that they contained sharpened, uneven, or serrated edges. These structural problems were due to imperfect finishing and polishing of these injection-molded implants. Choyce described[26,27] 17 Mark VIII style lenses that required removal because of UGH syndrome. He noted that these were actually poor copies of his original lens design, which had roughened edges as well. Choyce maintains that a well-maintained, properly sized implant of his design rarely causes these problems.[18] The incidence of this type of corrosion has declined dramatically with refinement of lens design and better control of manufacture of all lens edges. This syndrome still occurs occasionally in association with various types of modern implants, and it may very rarely occur following implantation of posterior chamber intra-ocular lenses as well.[28-31]

When an intra-ocular lens is noted to be causing an intra-ocular corrosion or erosion problem, the implant is best removed surgically immediately, with as little manipulation of the surrounding inflamed tissues as possible. Vitrectomy of the

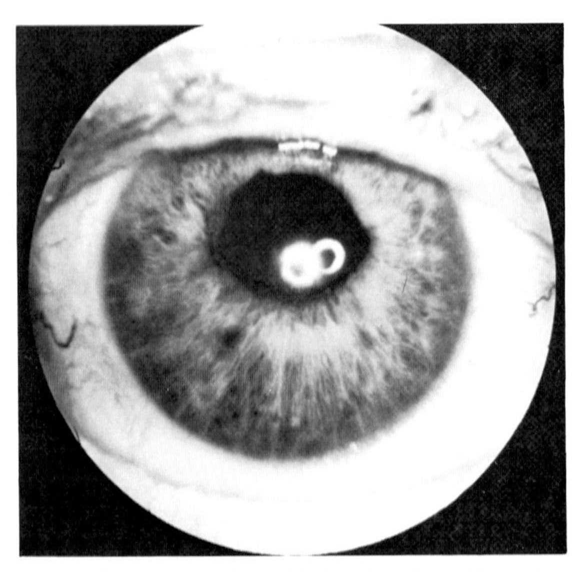

Figure 6-3. Patient with Fuchs' heterochromic cyclitis in whom cataract extraction was performed and posterior chamber intraocular lens was placed. Note the irregular pigmentary fallout and dispersion from the pupillary margin.

surrounding gel may be necessary, especially if the ongoing inflammation causes a "wick" syndrome leading to inflammatory cystoid macular edema. A posterior chamber lens, often fibrosed into position with its haptics securely in place, may have to have its haptics cut with firm scissors (often an intra-ocular foreign body scissors) in order to remove the optic from behind the pupil with minimal manipulation of the iris. If the offending structure is a haptic eroding through the iris stroma (see Fig. 6-2), a portion of the iris may have to be surgically cut or teased away in order to free the entrapped portion. An eye inflamed by the progressing and unrelenting tissue corrosion of intra-ocular lens-induced uveitis may necessitate a long period of recuperation, especially if cystoid macular edema had been present, and it should not be subjected to secondary lens implantation for a considerable time, if ever. Many of these eyes require at least 3 to 6 months for the keratic precipitates and the aqueous cell to disappear, and longer for the vitreous cell contents, debris, and "dusting" to clear (see Fig. 6-2). An even more prolonged recuperation may be necessary for the diminution of cystoid edema requiring repeated sub-Tenon injection of soluble steroid. Some few of these eyes never recuperate from the chronic cystoid edema even long after all signs of intra-ocular inflammation have disappeared.

Figure 6-3 demonstrates the profound degree of transillumination resulting from the prodigious iris stromal corrosion of this implant. Figure 6-4 demonstrates the inferior lens haptic of the posterior lens completely eroding through the iris stroma. Such examples of implant corrosion-induced uveitis demonstrate

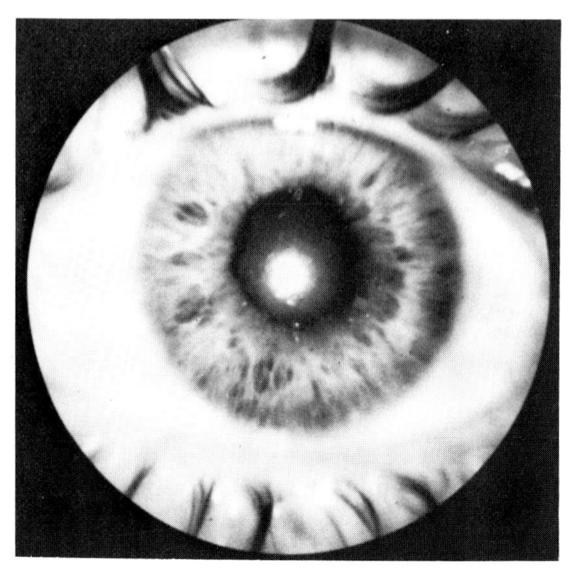

Figure 6-4. A 31-year-old man with Reiter's disease whose synechiae to his normal phakic lens were lysed using a YAG laser, being careful to place all of the fibrous cutting energy bursts on the anterior surface of the synechiae from the 8:00 to the 10:00 position.

the fact that no amount of steroid-applied immunosuppression is capable of reducing the uveitis in these eyes. Only surgical removal of the lenses will lead to the healing of the ocular structures involved.

Inflammation in the early postoperative period following intra-ocular lens

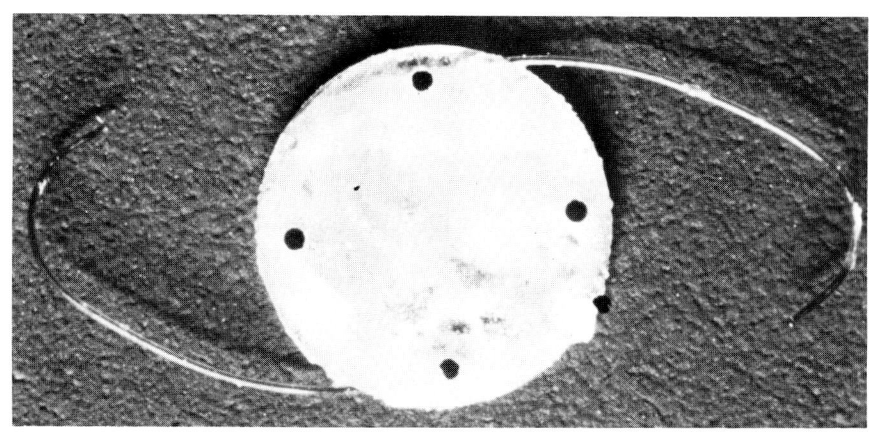

Figure 6-5. Intraocular lens removed from a patient. The entire anterior surface is coated with thick exudate. The lens served as a secondary cataract in a patient whose postoperative uveitic outpouring almost completely obscured the lens.

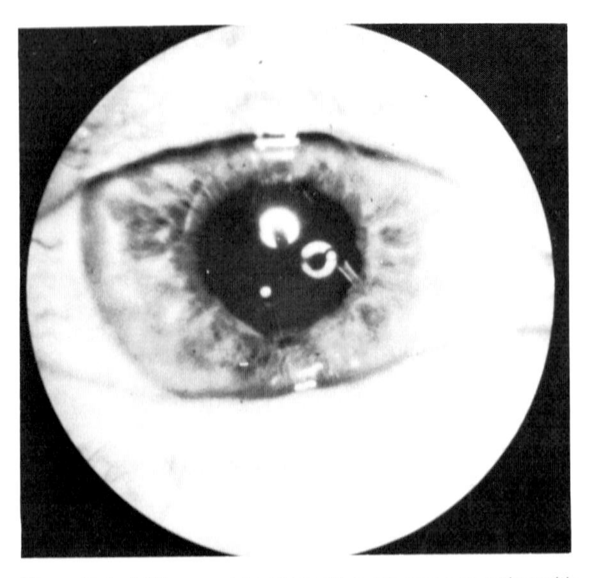

Figure 6-6. A 62-year-old patient after cataract extraction with posterior chamber lens implant who suffered iris bombé from total pupillary block secondary to uveitic scarring of pupillary margin to the implant. Note that these synechiae were successfully lysed at the 2:00, 4:00, and 8:00 positions using a YAG laser without disturbing the anterior surface of the implant itself.

implantation may, in part, be related to surgical manipulation occurring as a response to transient breakdown of the blood aqueous barrier, retained lens material following ECCE,[12,13,28] or tissue. Some surgeons have postulated an "immunologic" inflammation due to the implant material itself.[32–34] Some of this persistent intra-ocular type inflammation may be minimized or reduced by prostaglandin inhibitors, such as indomethacin or aspirin.[35,36] The retained lens material usually causes an inflammatory response that is transient and mild, and only in rare cases will it be prolonged or significant. The incidence of this type of transient iridocyclitis following extracapsular surgery has decreased markedly from the early days of intra-ocular lens implantation. However, one must always be mindful of the fact that the solution applied to the eye during surgery may have toxic elements and may even be contaminated. The report of Webster and co-workers represents the largest recognized series of fungal endophthalmitis due to contaminated intra-ocular lens neutralizing solutions, which was associated with intra-ocular lens implantation.[37,38]

Most studies have shown, however, that infectious endophthalmitis does not occur with higher frequency after IOL implantation than one might anticipate following simple cataract removal.[18,37,39–40] Several authors have reported infectious endophthalmitis,[18,37,38,42–44] done either to fungi or bacteria, associated with IOLs. Success of treatment varied in all of these reported cases, and while

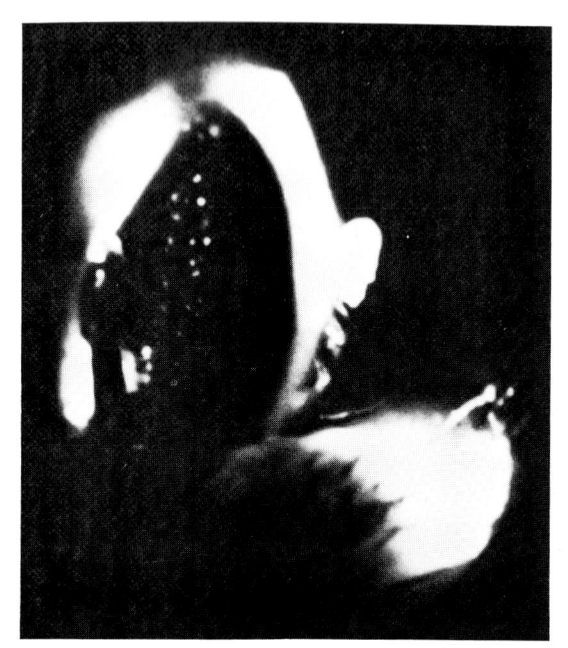

Figure 6-7. A 78-year-old patient, after cataract extraction, with anterior chamber lens implant eroding iris surface and causing an unremitting iridocyclitis in this patient. This intra-ocular lens-induced uveitis necessitated removal of the implant as a surgical cure.

removal of the implant was required in some situations,[43] in others the eye was treated successfully with the implant in place.[45]

Others

If inflammation is damaging to intra-ocular structures, such as the retina, cataract surgery will not noticeably affect the ultimate visual acuity. As in Behçet's syndrome or other forms of vasculitis, the optic nerve or retinal vasculature can be so damaged that cataract surgery may not improve vision. Conversely, it is stated that cataract extraction in cases of sympathetic ophthalmia is a benign procedure.

As noted, the less inflamed the eye, the better the prognosis for cataract surgery. For example, in a case of recurrent iridocyclitis that has been totally quiescent for several years, a routine cataract extraction can be performed without significant complications. But in cases of low-grade chronic inflammation with progressive cataract, a more judicious and cautious approach should be taken, especially if the cause cannot be determined or the syndrome identified. Intra-operative and postoperative corticosteroids are indicated in such cases.

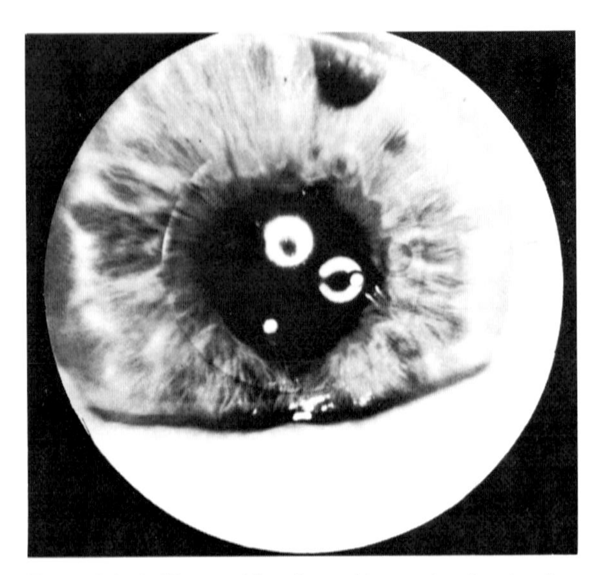

Figure 6-8. A 68-year-old patient with anterior chamber lens implant with intra-ocular lens-strut, which can be seen eroding through iris stroma causing an unremitting postoperative uveitis. This condition necessitated removal of the implant to alleviate intraocular inflammation.

General Approach and Surgical Management

If there is minimal or no active inflammation in an eye that has sustained previous bouts of inflammation, and if the patient is not receiving medication at the time of surgery, any standard lens extraction procedure can probably be performed without significant complications. In a young patient, careful extracapsular extraction is probably the safest procedure, if the pupil can be well dilated.

If there is chronic, active anterior segment inflammation with no posterior segment inflammation, including no vitreous cells or retinitis, an intense pre-operative therapeutic regimen of topical, sub-Tenon's capsule, and sometimes systemic corticosteroids is recommended for 7 to 10 days before surgery. The visual indications should be considered carefully in such cases because the risk of postoperative inflammation and other complications is not well documented. If extracapsular extractions are completed with great care, the removal of all lens material should be ensured. A well-dilated pupil is necessary.

If the inflammation is anterior and posterior, with cells and opacities in the vitreous, a combined lensectomy and vitrectomy is recommended, since residual inflammatory cells and debris in the vitreous cavity may increase the frequency with which the uveitis recurs. Diamond and Kaplan,[9,10] Nobe and co-workers,[15] Fitzgerald and co-workers,[16] and Belmont and Michelson[17] have reported various

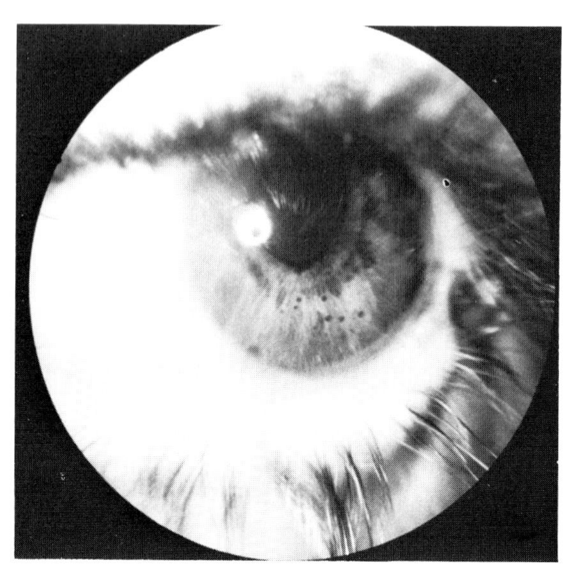

Figure 6-9. Eye with quieted inflammation after removal of the intraocular lens from intraocular lens–induced uveitis. Note that pigmented keratic precipitates persist long after the iridocyclitis of this lens-induced uveitis has subsided.

types of uveitis that respond well to lensectomy and vitrectomy. A pars plana approach is used with endo-illumination, standard vitrectomy-lensectomy techniques, and vitrectomy instrumentation (see Fig. 6-3). These techniques are also recommended for cases of juvenile rheumatoid arthritis, ankylosing spondylitis, and pars planitis with cataract.

Special Problems and Considerations

Synechiae

Synechiae may occur not only at the pupillary margin but also in the mid-periphery of the iris and between the ciliary process and the lens capsule. Whether intracapsular or extracapsular extraction is performed, gentle lysis of adhesions between the iris and lens is important. This can be performed in an iridotomy with instruments and gentle irrigation. During the intra-capsular extraction, slow and careful delivery of the lens should be accompanied by lysing of the remaining synechiae. Lensectomy-vitrectomy may be preferred in such cases.

Cyclitic Membrane

Patients with chronic uveitis, especially those with juvenile arthritis and persistent sarcoid uveitis, may have a cyclitic membrane extending from the ciliary body

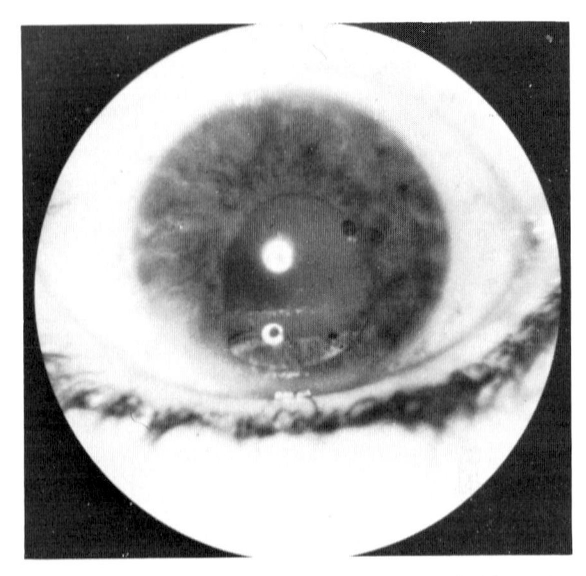

Figure 6-10. A 72-year-old patient whose superior iris capture and continuous excoriation by a posterior chamber lens caused unremitting iridocyclitis.

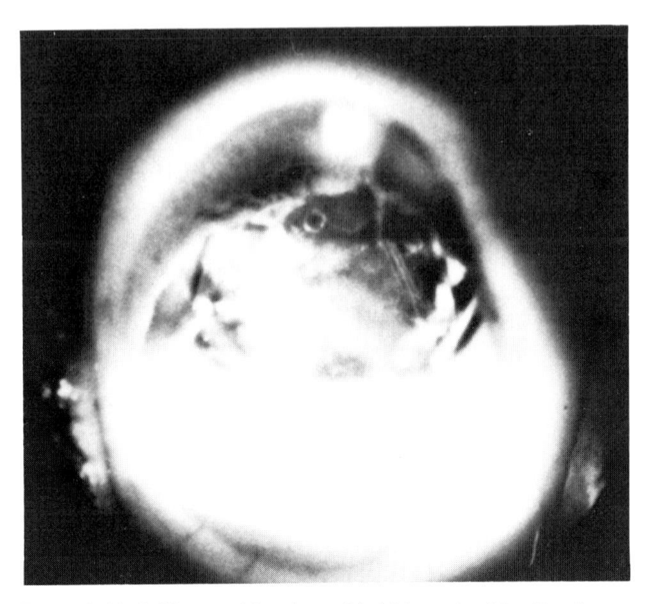

Figure 6-11. A 68-year-old patient with thickened, white, fibrotic posterior capsule secondary to intraocular, lens-induced iridocyclitis.

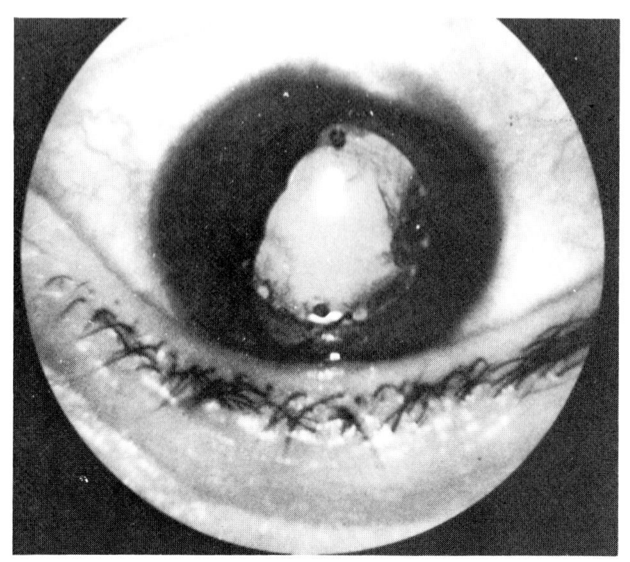

Figure 6-12. Same patient as in Fig. 6-11 after YAG capsulotomy; anterior segment quieted with steroids.

over the back surface of the lens (see Figs. 6-1 and 6-2). This membrane may be detected pre-operatively by ultrasonography. If a standard procedure with a large cataract section is to be carried out, the membrane should be excised with scissors in the pupillary zone only. In closed procedures in which endosurgical techniques are used, the membrane should be amputated along with the cataract and anterior vitreous. The surgeon must be prepared to deal with these membranes and remove as much of this tissue as possible during the cataract surgery. A cyclitic membrane that pulls on the ciliary body can cause its detachment, which in turn can lead to hypotony and phthisis. In aphakic eyes, some cyclitic membranes can be sectioned successfully with a yttrium-aluminum-garnet (YAG) laser (see Fig. 6-4), thus eliminating traction on the ciliary body. Usually the power needed is greatly in excess of a routine capsulotomy. Potentially, the YAG laser may be used to section the fibrous bands over the retina that lead to tractional retinal detachment.

Inflammatory Membrane Over the Surface of the Lens and Connected to the Iris

It is common for a membrane of vascularized connective tissue to extend from the iris over the entire pupillary area. Often this membrane can be separated mechanically from the iris and the anterior lens capsule. Transient bleeding that occurs during the removal of the membrane usually stops without causing significant problems. If the pupil can then be dilated, the surgeon can proceed with a routine cataract extraction.

Management of the Iris

A chronically inflamed iris tends to bleed easily during surgery, but the bleeding is often self-limited. In severe cases, bimanual, bipolar cautery must be used. Manipulation of the iris and surgery should be minimal.

In totally quiet eyes that have no tendency to develop synechiae, as in Fuch's heterochromic cyclitis or pars planitis, peripheral iridectomy may be satisfactory. However, if the case is more complicated and if a lens extraction is to be performed without vitrectomy, a sector iridectomy is safer. If a combined lensectomy-vitrectomy is performed, there can be no postoperative synechiae between the wound and the vitreous face or lens capsule, and pupillary block cannot develop. Iris surgery, therefore, is discouraged; not only can it contribute to postoperative inflammation, but it is unnecessary.

Vitreous Cells and Opacities

Ultrasonography in the pre-operative examination may reveal vitreous opacities. If these are extensive, a combined lensectomy and vitrectomy can be performed. However, if a standard lensectomy alone is planned, the vitreous face should be left intact, since its stability is thought to lessen the chance of cystoid macular edema.

The vitreous gel removed is laden with cellular elements, debris, and progressive architecture of fibrous material as a consequence of chronic uveitis, and is increasingly being appreciated to also contain "antigenic" substances that mediate or influence chronic or recurrent cystoid macular edema. Thus, it is felt by some specialists that cataract extraction with subtotal vitrectomy (pars plana approach), being careful to maintain the posterior lens capsule, helps, in part, to improve and stabilize visual acuity by reducing macular edema. While the fluorescein angiographic appearance might not appreciably change, the vision loss from that macula often improves appreciably. In other instances, the edema is reduced dramatically after removal of debris-laden gel. While it is clinically accepted that a significant clouding of the vitreous (either through hemorrhage or cellular infiltration) may cause surprisingly little diminution of vision (i.e., almost no retina detail "viewed" with patient vision of 20/50 or so), it is of genuine interest how much vision is regained after removal of the clouded "antigenic" gel (i.e., a vision of counting fingers to 20/200 may improve to 20/200 and to 20/40 respectively).

Intra-ocular Lenses in Uveitis Patients

To date, there is limited experience with intra-ocular lenses which have been implanted after cataract extraction in uveitis patients. Most surgeons believe that intra-ocular lenses are an added and unnecessary hazard for patients who already have had intra-ocular inflammation. Therefore, at this time intra-ocular lenses are not recommended after cataract surgery in patients with uveitis. Special situations are now being considered in which posterior chamber lenses are being implanted specifically "in the bag." The surgeon in these experimental situations specifies that the presence of the lens will probably have little or no influence on the initiation or recurrence of intra-ocular inflammation.[46] One common sequela of IOLs in this situation is the accumulation of keratitic precipitates and debris on the surface of the implant which tends to reduce vision minimally.

Intra-ocular lenses, however, are a well-established, modern-day etiology for a smoldering, intractable uveitis resulting from disruption, irritation, or corrosion of uveal tissue (Fig. 6-5, 6-6). The only cure for such an "irritative" uveitis is removal of the intra-ocular lens. A special clinical presentation of the old, rigid, larger lens was the UGH syndrome, in which the inter-related findings of uveitis, glaucoma, and hyphema were coincident, necessitating removal of the offending implant (Fig. 6-7).

References

1. Schlaegel TF Jr: Essentials of Uveitis, chap 4–12. Boston, Little, Brown & Company, 1969
2. Ridley H: Cataract surgery in chronic uveitis. Trans Ophthalmol Soc UK 85:519, 1965
3. Key SN III, Kimura SJ: Iridocyclitis associated with juvenile rheumatoid arthritis. Am J Ophthalmol 80:425, 1975
4. Ward DM, Hart CT: Complicated cataract extraction in Fuchs' heterochromic uveitis. Br J Ophthalmol 51:530, 1967
5. Norn MS: Cataract extraction in Fuchs' heterochromia. Acta Ophthalmol 46:685, 1968
6. Smith RE, O'Connor GR: Cataract extraction in Fuchs' syndrome. Arch Ophthalmol 91:39, 1974
7. Liesengang TJ: Clinical features and prognosis in Fuchs' uveitis syndrome. Arch Ophthalmol 100:1622, 1982
8. Smith RE, Godfrey WA, Kimura SJ: Complications of chronic cyclitis. Am J Ophthalmol 82:277, 1976
9. Diamond JG, Kaplan HJ: Lensectomy and vitrectomy for complicated cataract secondary to uveitis. Arch Ophthalmol 96:1798, 1978
10. Diamond JG, Kaplan HJ: Uveitis: Effect of vitrectomy combined with lensectomy. Ophthalmology 86:1320, 1979
11. Wirostko E, Spalter HF: Lens induced uveitis. Arch Ophthalmol 78:1, 1967
12. Riise P: Endophthalmitis phacoanaphylactica. Am J Ophthalmol 60:911, 1965
13. Easom HA, Zimmerman LE: Sympathetic ophthalmia and bilateral phacoanaphylaxis. Arch Ophthalmol 72:9, 1964
14. deVeer JA: Bilateral endophthalmitis phacoanaphylactica. Arch Ophthalmol 49:607, 1953

15. Nobe JR, Kokoris N, Diddie KR et al: Lensectomy-vitrectomy in chronic uveitis. Retina 3:71, 1983
16. Fitzgerald CR: Pars plana vitrectomy for vitreous opacity secondary to presumed toxoplasmosis. Arch Ophthalmol 98:321, 1980
17. Belmont JB, Michelson JB: Vitrectomy in uveitis associated with ankylosing spondylitis. Am J Ophthalmol 94:300, 1982
18. Apple DJ, Mamalis N, Steinmetz RL et al: Phacoanaphylactic endophthalmitis associated with ECCE and posterior chamber IOL. Arch Ophthalmol (in press)
19. Apple DJ, Rabb MR: Clinical Applications of Ocular Pathology, 3rd ed. St Louis, CV Mosby, 1985
20. Hogan MJ, Zimmerman LE: Ophthalmic Pathology, pp 153–156. Philadelphia, WB Saunders, 1962
21. Rahi AHS, Garner A: Immunopathology of the Eye, pp 204–220. Oxford, Blackwell Scientific Publications, 1976
22. Perlman EM, Albert DM: Clinically unsuspected phacoanaphylaxis after ocular trauma. Arch Ophthalmol 95:144–146, 1977
23. Ellingson FT: Complications with the Choyce Mark VII anterior chamber lens implant (uveitis-glaucoma-hyphema). Am Intra-Ocular Implant Soc J 3:199–205, 1977
24. Ellingson FT: The uveitis-glaucoma-hyphema syndrome associated with the Mark VIII anterior chamber lens implant. Am Intra-Ocular Implant Soc J 4:50–53, 1978
25. Keates RH, Ehrlich DR: "Lenses of chance" complications of anterior chamber implants. Ophthalmology 85:408–414, 1978
26. Choyce DP: Complications of the AC implants of the early 1950's and the UGH or Ellingson syndrome of the late 1970's. Am Intra-Ocular Implant Soc J 4:22, 1978
27. Choyce DP: Anterior chamber implants—Past, present, and future. The VIth Binkhorst medal lecture. Am Intra-Ocular Implant Soc J 8:42–50, 1982
28. Beehler ME: Letter: UGH syndrome with the 91-Z lens. Am Intra-Ocular Implant Soc J 9:459, 1983
29. Ambache H, Kavanagh L, Whiting J: Effect of mechanical stimulation on rabbits' eyes: Release of active substances in anterior chamber perfusates. J Physiol (London) 176:378–384, 1965
30. Lucas DR: Scanning electron microscopy of intraocular lenses. In Rosen ES, Haining WM, Arnott EJ (eds): Intraocular Lens Implantation, pp 583–591. St Louis, CV Mosby, 1984
31. Percival SP, Das SK: UGH syndrome after posterior chamber lens implantation. Am Intra-Ocular Implant Soc J 9:200–201, 1983
32. Binkhorst CD: Ridley's intraocular lens prosthesis: The postoperative reaction. Results obtained in 12 cases. Ophthalmologica 133:383–392, 1957
33. Binkhorst CD: Iris-supported artificial pseudophakia. A new development in intraocular artificial lens surgery (iris clip lens). Trans Ophthalmol Soc UK 79:469–584, 1959
34. Binkhorst CD: Results of implantation of intraocular lenses in unilateral aphakia. With special reference to the pupillary or iris clip lens—A new method of fixation. Am J Ophthalmol 49:703–710, 1960
35. Jampol LM, Sanders DR, Kraff MC: Prophylaxis and therapy of aphakic cystoid macular edema. Surv Ophthalmol (Suppl)28:535–539, 1984

36. Kraff MC, Sanders DR, Jampol LM et al: Prophylaxis of pseudophakic cystoid macular edema with topical indomethacin. Ophthalmology 89:885–890, 1982
37. Mosier MA, Lusk B, Pettit TH et al: Fungal endophthalmitis following intraocular lens implantation. Am J Ophthalmol 83:1–8, 1977
38. Pettit TH, Olson RJ, Foos RY et al: Fungal endophthalmitis following intraocular lens implantation: a surgical epidemic. Arch Ophthalmol 98:1025–1039, 1980
39. Drews RC: Inflammatory response, endophthalmitis, corneal dystrophy, glaucoma, retinal detachment, dislocation, refractive error, lens removal and enucleation. Ophthalmology 85:164–175, 1978
40. Emery JM, McIntyre DJH: Extracapsular Cataract Surgery, pp 1–418. St Louis, CV Mosby, 1983
41. Stark WJ, Worthern DM, Holladay JR et al: The FDA report on intraocular lenses. Ophthalmology 90:311–317, 1983
42. Nirankari VS, Karesh JW, Lakhampal V et al: Pseudophakic endophthalmitis. Ophthalmic Surg 14:314–316, 1983
43. Gerding DN, Poley B, Hall WH et al: Treatment of pseudomonas endophthalmitis associated with prosthetic intraocular lens implantation. Am J Ophthalmol 88:902–908, 1979
44. Galin MA: Causes of implant inflammation. In Rosen ES, Haining WM, Arnott EJ (eds): Intraocular Lens Implantation, pp 563–565. St Louis, CV Mosby, 1984
45. Petrilli AM, Balfort R, Abram MT et al: Ultrasonic fragmentation of cataract in uveitis. Retina 2:61–65, 1986
46. Weinberg R: IOL implantation in patients with intraocular inflammation. San Francisco, American Academy of Ophthalmologists Annual Meeting, 1985

SEVEN

Vitrectomy

At present, the indication for vitrectomy in cases of intra-ocular inflammation is twofold. It is used as a controlled biopsy of the vitreous to establish the histologic diagnosis of endophthalmitis (Fig. 7-1); large cell lymphoma (reticulum cell sarcoma; Fig. 7-2), and other unusual infiltrations of the vitreous (Table 7-1; Figs. 7-3, 7-4, and 7-5). It also serves as a therapeutic intervention in many cases (Figs. 7-6 and 7-7). Combined lensectomy-vitrectomy has not resulted in a worsening of the inflammation of phthisis.

Diagnostic Vitrectomy

Certain forms of ocular inflammation lend themselves to diagnostic vitrectomy.[1] Patients with large cell lymphoma (reticulum cell sarcoma) are usually elderly and have bilateral chronic inflammation with a predominance of cells in the vitreous cavity[2,3] and thus are suspected of having reticulum cell sarcoma. Since the treatment of this disease requires irradiation to the eye as well as the brain (Figs. 7-8, 7-9), and chemotherapy or both and *not* corticosteroids, a diagnostic vitrectomy, performed with a standard pars plana technique, is recommended (see Fig. 7-2). The vitreous specimens should be collected and taken immediately to a cytology laboratory. Handling of the intra-ocular specimens by the pathology or cytology division should be planned in advance. If possible, the specimen should

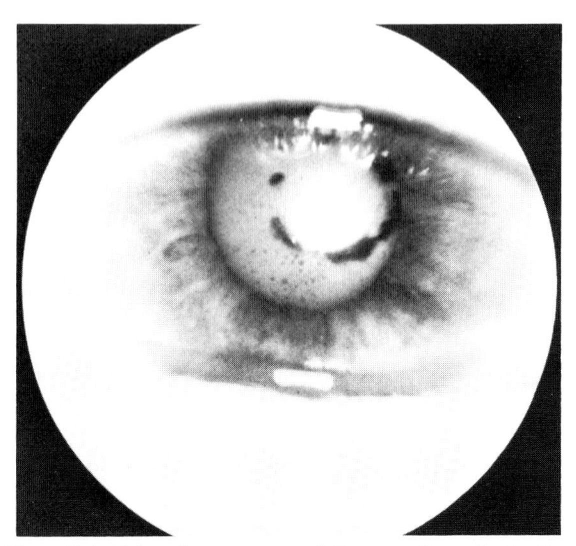

Figure 7-1. External appearance of the eye of a patient with Vogt-Koyanagi-Harada disease and chronic thickened vitreous, which gives the gross appearance of a cataract through a clear lens. Note the large mutton fat precipitates and pigment ring on the anterior lens capsule.

be obtained by aspiration alone, since vitreous cutters can distort the cells. These patients often have a "fluid" vitreous, which makes aspiration feasible and extensive cutting unnecessary. These cells can then be examined both histologically and for their surface immunoglobulins.[1,4] Other types of metastatic cancer cells such as adenocarcinoma, breast carcinoma, acute and chronic lymphocytic leukemia, and metastatic malignant melanoma[1,4,5] can be found in the vitreous in unusual cases.

Diagnostic vitrectomy also may be indicated in young patients presumed to have *Toxocara canis* endophthalmitis and in patients suspected of having infectious endophthalmitis, especially of fungal origin. Numerous eosinophils may be seen with *Toxocara* in the vitreous aspirate and an enzyme-linked immunosorbent assay (ELISA) should be performed on the specimen. In fungal endophthalmitis, hyphae and yeast forms may be identified.

Lensectomy should be avoided if a diagnostic vitrectomy is being performed; the lens is usually clear in such cases, and a mixture of lens material and vitreous contents may be very confusing to the cytologist.

The approach to suspected infectious endophthalmitis is controversial. While it is generally accepted that immediate aqueous and vitreous taps for cultures and smears are important first steps, and that topical, subconjunctival, and parenteral antibiotics are necessary, the role of intravitreal antibiotics and of therapeutic vitrectomy is less well defined.[6-13] We feel that intravitreal antibiotics are indicated in most cases of suspected bacterial endophthalmitis and that these

TABLE 7-1. Diagnostic Paracentesis: Findings

Finding	Condition or Disease Indicated
Aqueous	
Bacteria	Endophthalmitis
Fungi	*Candida, Aspergillus,* etc.
Tumor cells	Retinoblastoma, malignant melanoma, reticulum cell sarcoma, leukemia, metastatic cancer
Eosinophils	*Toxocara canis*
Macrophages	Phakolytic glaucoma
Antibodies (ELISA)	*Toxoplasma gondii, Toxocara canis,* Reticulum cell sarcoma, Behçet's disease, syphilis
Immune complexes	Behçet's disease
Other proteins	
Angiotensin-converting enzymes	Sarcoid
Lactate dehydrogenase isoenzyme	Retinoblastoma
Vitreous	
Bacteria	Endophthalmitis
Fungi	*Candida, Aspergillus,* etc.
Tumor cells	Retinoblastoma, malignant melanoma, reticulum cell sarcoma, leukemia
Eosinophils	*Toxocara canis*
Antibodies	*Toxoplasma gondii,* reticulum cell sarcoma, Behçet's disease, syphilis (and immune complexes)
Macrophages	Sympathetic ophthalmia, severe retinitis

can be injected during aqueous and vitreous paracentesis. There is, likewise, some general agreement that if marked vitreous exudation obscures the retinal vasculature (indirect ophthalmoscopy), therapeutic vitrectomy is indicated (see Figs. 7-2, 7-3, 7-5). If the retina can be easily visualized with minimal vitreous reaction, it is probably safer to treat the patient with subconjunctival, parenteral, and intravitreal antibiotics (such patients may have Staphylococcus epidermidis, which does well without vitrectomy) and to follow him closely. If the disease progresses and there is further clouding of the vitreous, we recommend immediate vitrectomy.

Vitrectomy may also allow medications to penetrate more deeply, since the surgical intervention further disrupts the blood-retinal barrier. The possibility of a retinal toxic reaction to medications is greater during and after vitrectomy, since the medication contacts the retina more directly. Therefore, more dilute solutions of a drug should be used during and after the vitrectomy procedure than before it. This is especially true in the use of amphotericin B and intra-ocular antibiotics.

Technically, a total vitrectomy may not be necessary and a "core" vitrectomy may suffice. The inflammatory membranes that result from endophthal-

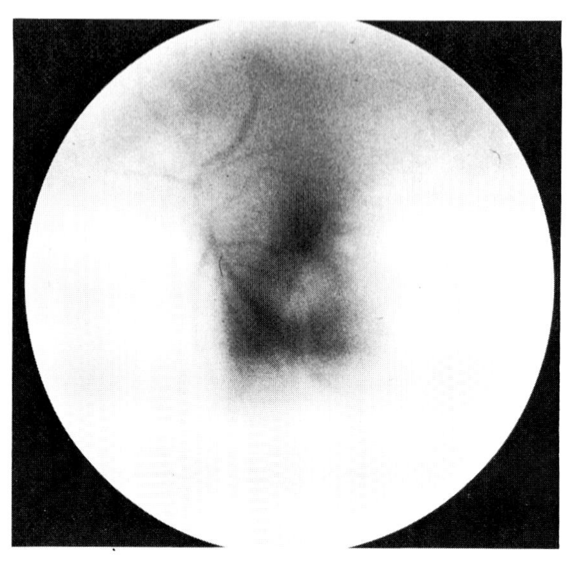

Figure 7-2. Pre-operative view of the fundus demonstrates chronic thick exudate in the vitreous gel, obscuring the view of the retina.

mitis often adhere tightly to the retina (see Figs. 7-5, 7-6), and a total vitrectomy can severely damage the retina, although it may be necessary to peel these membranes during vitrectomy.

If bacterial endophthalmitis is associated with an implanted lens, it is not always necessary to remove the lens. During a "closed" vitrectomy, the inflammatory membranes in the anterior chamber can be removed through an anterior incision, and the vitrectomy can be performed at the same time through the pars plana. The implant should probably be removed in cases of suspected fungal endophthalmitis.

Therapeutic Vitrectomy

There is increasing evidence that vitrectomy is of therapeutic value in various uveitic syndromes, both to eliminate the "burden" of inflammatory debris, threatening fibrous bands, and chronic opacification in the vitreous, as well as to ameliorate the macular edema, which is thought to be related to the vitreous and retinal inflammation (see Figs. 7-1, 7-2, 7-6, and 7-7). Diamond and Kaplan[14,15] found that the cystoid maculopathy that was present in most of their patients gradually resolved in the course of a year or more with remarkable return of vision. Belmont and Michelson[16] reported similar results in patients with chronic vitreal infiltration from ankylosing spondylitis. If there is an advanced cataract for any occlusion of the pupillary space in a patient with coexisting intra-ocular, predominantly vitreal, inflammation, a combined lensectomy and vitrectomy is practicable. Specifically, patients with chronic uveitis and dense cataract or nonspecific indolent posterior inflammation and cataract are candidates for this

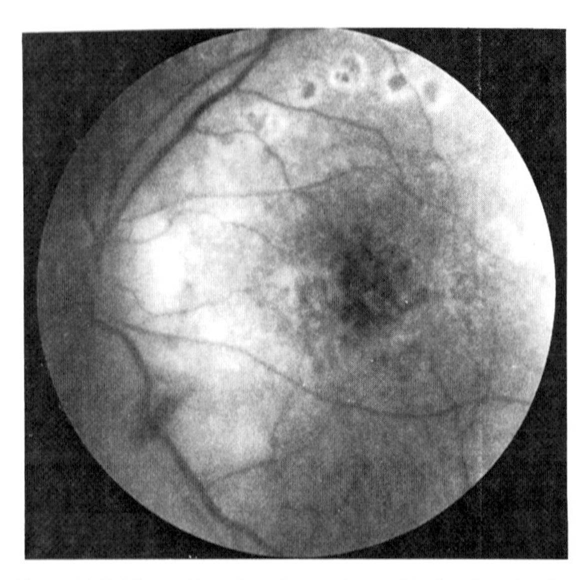

Figure 7-3. View after vitrectomy shows the fundus clearly. Note argon laser scars superotemporal to the optic disc, resulting from a previous laser treatment administered by an ophthalmologist for a serous retinal detachment.

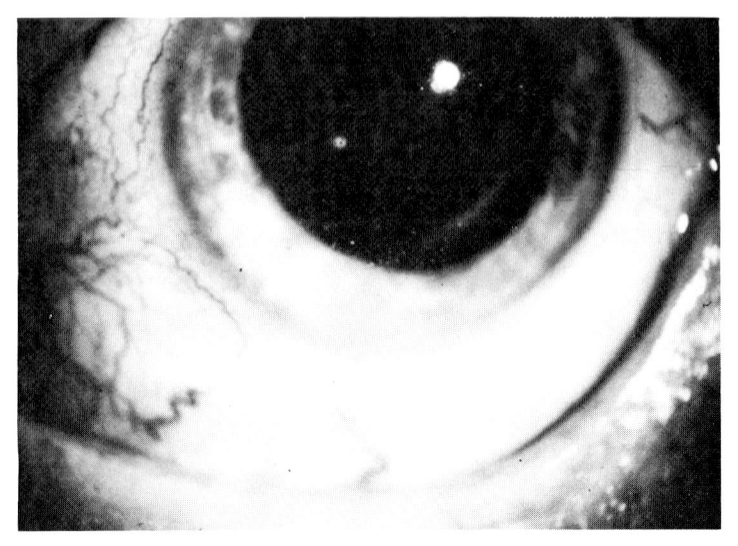

Figure 7-4. External view of the eye of a 76-year-old man in whom reticulum cell sarcoma (large cell lymphoma) is suspected. Note large mutton fat keratic precipitates.

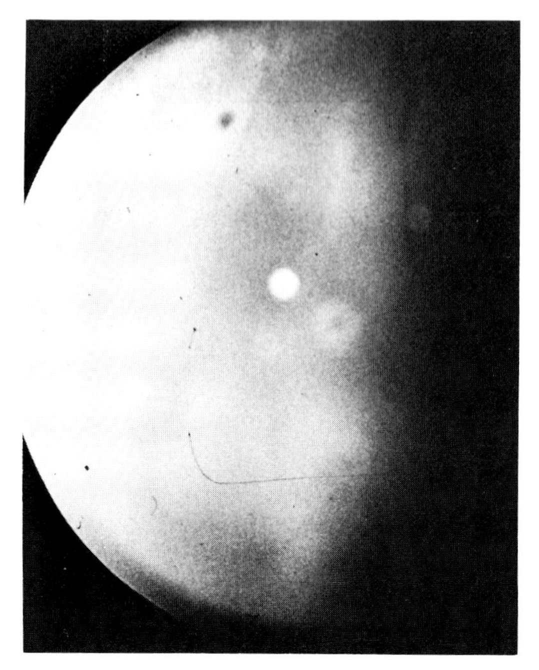

Figure 7-5. Fundus view of the patient in Figure 7-4 demonstrates 3+ vitreous cells and white subretinal infiltration.

procedure. Diamond and Kaplan[14,15] have reported that these patients tolerate lensectomy-vitrectomy well, and there seems to be no increased incidence of postoperative inflammation, phthisis, or other complications that have been regularly associated with standard cataract extraction in patients with uveitis.

Indications

What we currently consider an indication for lensectomy-vitrectomy in patients with intra-ocular inflammation is the presence of at least two of the following:

1. Need for better vision
2. Progressive disease (hypotony, premonitory signs of phthisis, especially in the presence of cyclitic membrane)
3. Complications requiring surgery (e.g., retinal detachment, tractional or rhegmatogenous)
4. Iris bombé (closed angle with synechiae) with hypotony (indicating the presence of a cyclitic membrane)

Technicalities

It is very important to assess the visual function of these patients before surgery. An electroretinogram (ERG) and the visual evoked potential (VEP) are important

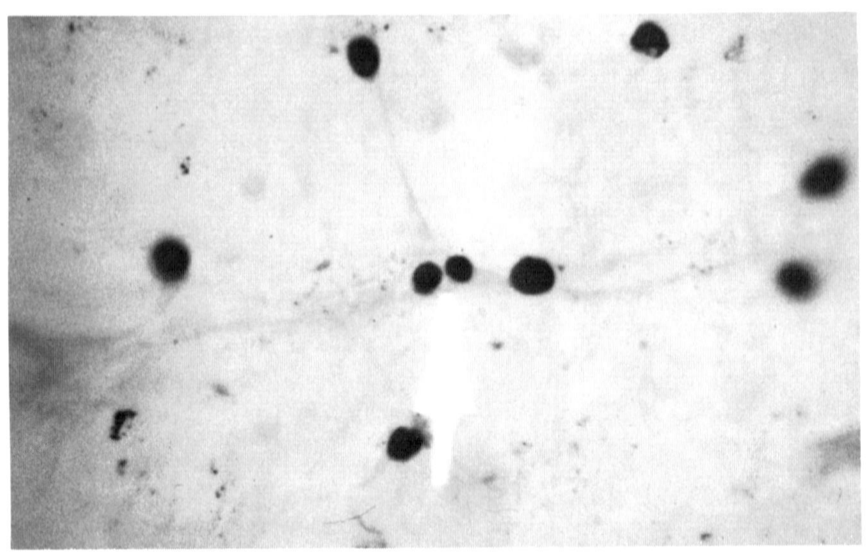

Figure 7-6. Vitreous aspirate demonstrates large cell lymphoma infiltrate. Note two smaller cells in mitosis (*arrow*).

to determine the condition of the retina and optic nerve; ultrasonography, particularly of the anterior segment, is helpful in determining whether there is thickening of the choroid or a cyclitic membrane that could create significant problems at the time of surgery. A thickened choroid suggests engorgement of choroidal vessels, and the presence of a cyclitic membrane may make penetration of the

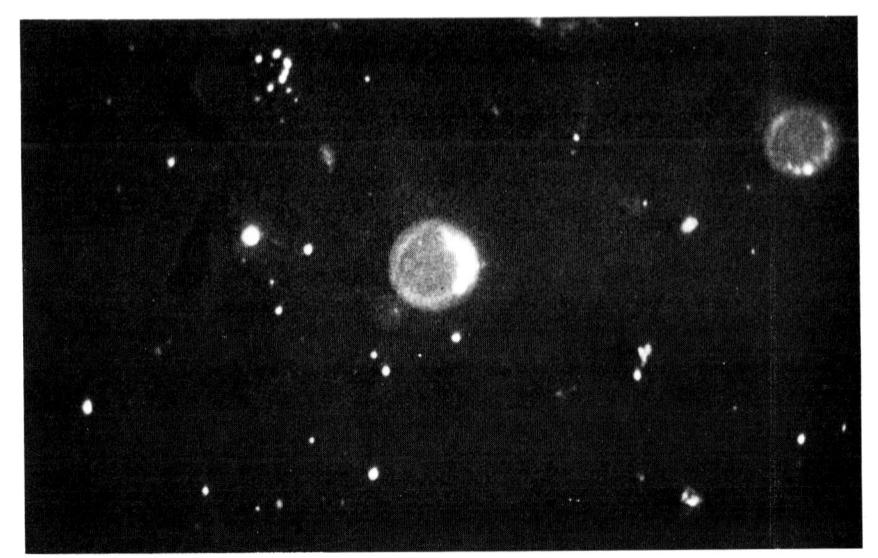

Figure 7-7. Vitreous cells stained for surface immunoglobulin light chains. Fluorescein discloses IgM light chains only as a corroboration of the monoclonal nature of this malignant infiltration.

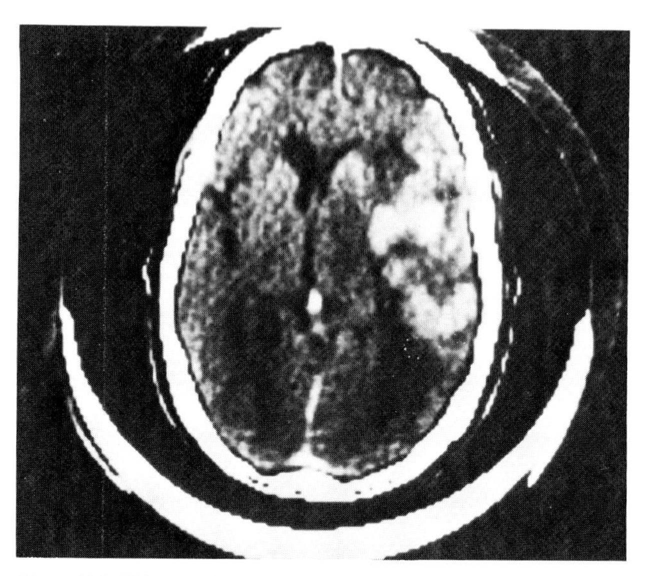

Figure 7-8. CT scan of the patient in Figure 7-4 (different time) shows intracerebral microgliomatosis of large cell lymphoma infiltration.

pars plana area difficult and complications such as hemorrhage or dialysis more likely.

If the eye is hypotonous prior to surgery, a cyclitic membrane is probably present even if it cannot be detected by ultrasonography (Figs. 7-10, 7-11). If there is a thickened choroid or a cyclitic membrane, a longer infusion cannula should be used in the pars plana area, and it is wise to remove as much of the lens as possible before turning on the posterior infusion cannula. In this way one can be reasonably certain that the cannula is through the pars plana and the cyclitic membrane. Lensectomy can be performed through the pars plana stab incisions with the infusion needle in one side of the lens and the vitrectomy instrument in the other side.

Synechiae should be removed or broken very early. If synechiae are dense, as in patients with juvenile rheumatoid arthritis, sarcoid, or ankylosing spondylitis, a stab incision should be made through the limbus. The synechiae should then be broken with a cyclodialysis spatula or other instrument to allow dilatation of the pupil, which facilitates the surgical procedure.

A subtotal vitrectomy is important in most cases, but attempts to remove the very organized vitreous at the vitreous base may result in an unnecessary "tug" on the peripheral retina.

Too aggressive a vitrectomy and repeated unnecessary peripheral manipulation can often result in retinal tears, which, combined with the underlying inflammatory disorder, eventuate in proliferative vitreoretinopathy (PVR or MPP) with subretinal membrane growth. One should perform a core vitrectomy to the optic nerve and employ sweeping gestures to remove cortical vitreous in the anteropos-

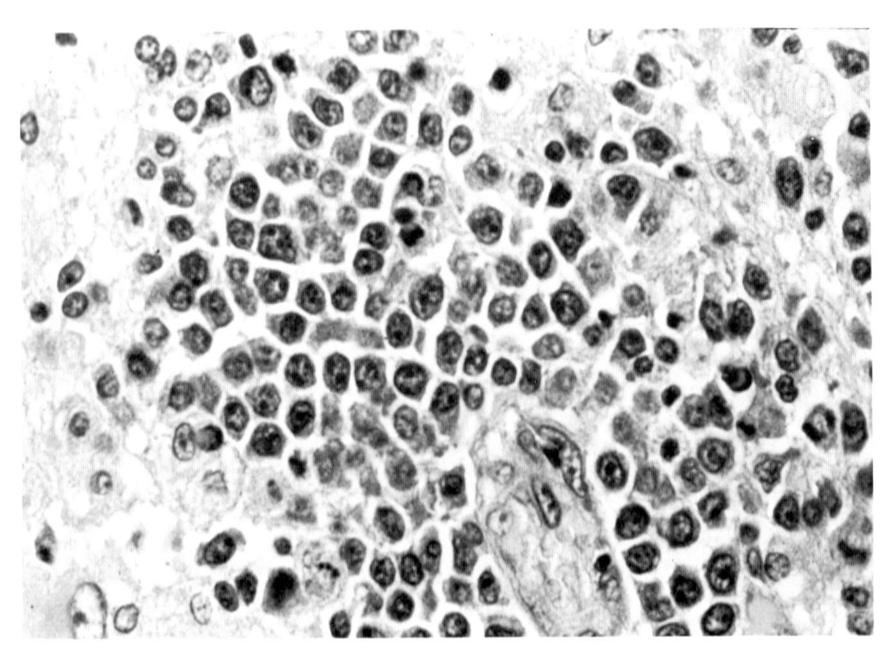

Figure 7-9. Histologic appearance of this brain tumor of "reticulum cell sarcoma" or large cell lymphoma.

terior direction. The peripheral "coring" procedure should be carried only slightly past the equator, with careful consideration given to avoid "tugging." One must remember that vitreous condensation and band formation are the rule, especially with endophthalmitis, and large expanses of vitreoretinal adhesion are common even in the posterior pole.

A peripheral "skirt" of dense vitreous does not appear to be a significant postoperative problem and can be left in place. Careful indirect ophthalmoscopy and scleral depression at the close of the procedure are indicated to detect dialysis and retinal tears. Cryopexy or scleral buckling procedures can be performed at this time.

The use of systemic, subconjunctival, and topical corticosteroids pre-operatively and sub-Tenon's capsule and systemic and topical corticosteroids postoperatively is recommended. Any retinal complications should be repaired at the time of vitrectomy.

Many reports describe the use of vitrectomy to remove vitreous opacities secondary to ocular inflammatory disease.[14–23] Fitzgerald successfully used pars plana vitrectomy and lensectomy in several patients with presumed ocular toxoplasmosis.[18] Diamond and Kaplan performed combined lensectomy and vitrectomy on 15 eyes of 13 patients who had acute recurrent or chronic uveitis.[14,15] Although visual improvement was noted in every eye in the latter series, maximal improvement was often limited by cystoid macular edema. Only one of the 15 eyes in the Diamond and Kaplan series had uveitis associated with ankylosing

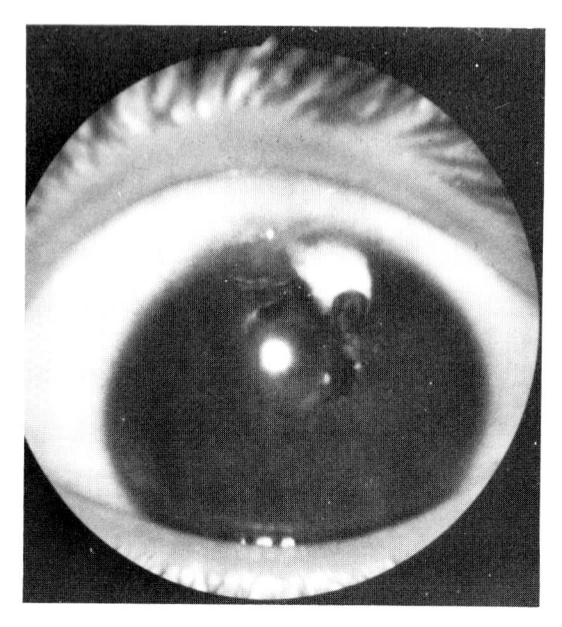

Figure 7-10. A 26-year-old aphakic white girl with juvenile rheumatoid arthritis. Photograph demonstrates updrawn fibrotic pupil with dense cyclitic membrane in a hypotonous eye.

spondylitis. Preoperative visual acuity in this eye was light perception. After combined lensectomy and vitrectomy, the visual acuity improved to 20/400 but remained limited by persistent optic nerve edema and macular pucker.

Vitreous opacification may occur in recurrent iridocyclitis as a consequence of posterior spillover of inflammatory cells, fibrin, and other materials from the ciliary body into the vitreous.[24-26] After a single episode of iridocyclitis, inflammatory cells in the vitreous may persist for months before clearing.[27] When slow clearance of inflammatory cells from the vitreous is combined with chronic iridocyclitis, progressive vitreous opacification may occur.[14]

The complex structural network of normal vitreous collagen provides an ideal scaffolding for accumulation and persistence of various cellular and organic mediators of acute and chronic inflammation. Many cell types may subsequently contribute to the formation of vitreous opacities, including fibrous astrocytes, fibrocytes, myofibroblasts, macrophages, various types of inflammatory cells, and hyalocytes.[28] Although hyalocyte participation in vitreous collagen synthesis is known to occur,[29-32] formation of collagenous vitreous opacities may actually result from participation of any or all of these cell types.[28]

Our own patients have demonstrated that, in chronic recurrent iridocyclitis, accumulation of inflammatory cells and materials within the vitreous may lead to vitreous opacification that interferes with vision.

Chronic recurrent iridocyclitis of various etiologies may be associated with a spillover of inflammatory cells into the vitreous cavity. If allowed to continue,

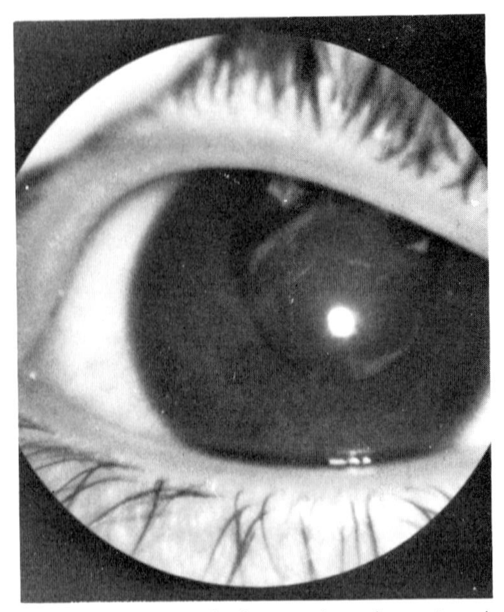

Figure 7-11. After pupiloplasty and membranectomy/ vitrectomy, a large round pupil is restored along with normal ocular tension. Vision improved from counting fingers to 20/40 plus with contact lens. The ocular pressure increased, also, due to removal of traction from cyclitic membrane on the ciliary body, which then restored its more normal secretory function.

this can lead to gross vitreous opacification, which prevents clear visualization of posterior segment structures. Even in aphakic eyes, the scaffolding provided by the intact vitreous proves sufficient for chronic vitreous opacification to occur.

By removing the scaffolding previously provided by formed vitreous, inflammatory cells and materials entering the posterior segment through the ciliary body are free to circulate to routes of egress in the anterior segment. Despite continued chronic iridocyclitis, the vitreous cavity can often remain optically clear after vitrectomy for a long period of time.

Ocular inflammation in these eyes is usually not exacerbated by surgical intervention. Periocular administration of an intermediate-acting corticosteroid immediately before surgery often prevents postsurgical inflammation. Although chronic low-grade iridocyclitis and cystoid macular edema prevent maximum visual recovery in most of these instances, vitrectomy may result in stable visual improvement.

The posterior spillover of inflammatory materials in chronic iridocyclitis associated with ankylosing spondylitis and Reiter's disease may result in persistent vitreous opacification. Previous reports seem to overlook this finding, describing the uveitis associated with ankylosing spondylitis as "acute," "intermittent," and "anterior" in nature.[4,8,33,34] When iridocyclitis associated with ankylosing spondylitis becomes chronic, the cumulative effects of secondary involvement of the vitreous may result in visually disabling vitreous debris and opacification, making affected eyes good candidates for vitrectomy. Although vitrectomy must be chosen only after prolonged follow-up and careful consideration, it appears to offer a definite increase in vision in certain cases.

Because of the intense episodes of recurrent inflammation, it is essential to render these eyes as quiet as possible before an operation by means of topical, peri-ocular, or systemic corticosteroids. Diamond and Kaplan attribute much of their success to the minimal degree of inflammation present in the eyes at time of surgery. Pre-operative ultrasound is also helpful in determining the degree of vitreous opacification, thickening of the choroid, and the presence of a cyclitic membrane, which can create significant technical problems at surgery.

The major objective of surgery in these patients with complication uveitic cataract and vitreous opacification is to improve vision. Our own experience[16] compares favorably with the visual results reported by others (Diamond and Kaplan,[14,15] Kanski,[36] Fitzgerald,[18] Nobe and co-workers[17]).

Vitrectomy may modify the dynamics of the uveitic process favorably. Although lensectomy-vitrectomy does not reduce the inflammatory reaction in all cases, Diamond and Kaplan state that their patients noted a subjective decrease in the severity of recurrent episodes in the operated eye.[14] Kanski[36] presented a series of 77 cases of juvenile rheumatoid arthritis with uveitis and cataract treated with lensectomy and partial anterior vitrectomy. In Kanski's patients, who probably represent a very poor risk category, there was improvement in vision but no marked improvement in the course of the uveitis.

Cystoid macular edema was the major cause of decreased visual acuity after operation, although this is a common and serious complication of chronic uveitis even without surgery.[14,15,20,24,37] In our own series, most eyes with postoperative cystoid macular edema had this complication at the time of surgery, as observed with the operating microscope. One case of cystoid macular edema resolved spontaneously several months after surgery.

Diamond and Kaplan[14] suggested that vitrectomy may reduce cystoid macular edema and reported gradual resolution over the course of a year, with considerable improvement in vision in some patients. Federman[37] reported complete resolution of cystoid macular edema in 20 of 22 patients who underwent vitrectomy for vitreous adhesions to the wound with persistent Irvine-Gass syndrome associated with mild vitreous inflammation. However, vitrectomy itself is a rare "cause" of cystoid macular edema.[38] Other complications observed are similar to known complications of cataract surgery, lensectomy, and vitrectomy.[39–41]

References

1. Engel HM, Green WR, Michels RG et al: Diagnostic vitrectomy. Retina 1:121, 1981

2. Michelson JB, Michelson PE, Bordin GM et al: Ocular reticulum cell sarcoma: Presentation as retinal detachment with demonstration of monoclonal immunoglobulin light chains on the vitreous cells. Arch Ophthalmol 99:1409, 1981
3. Char DH: Immunology of Uveitis and Ocular Tumors. New York, Grune & Stratton, 1978
4. Michelson JB: Color Atlas of Uveitis Diagnosis. Chicago, Year Book Medical Publishers, 1984
5. Robertson DM, Wilkinson CP, Murray JL et al: Metastatic tumor to the retina and vitreous cavity from primary melanoma of the skin. Ophthalmology 88:1296, 1981
6. Cottingham AJ Jr, Foster RK: Vitrectomy in endophthalmitis: Results of study using vitrectomy, intraocular antibiotics, or a combination of both. Arch Ophthalmol 94:2078, 1978
7. Eichenbaum DM, Jaffe NS, Clayman HM et al: Pars plana vitrectomy as a primary treatment for acute bacterial endophthalmitis. Am J Ophthalmol 86:167, 1978
8. Forster RK: Etiology and diagnosis of bacterial postoperative endophthalmitis. Ophthalmology Otolaryngol 85:320, 1978
9. Forster RK, Zachary IG, Cottingham AJ Jr et al: Further observations on the diagnosis, cause, and treatment of endophthalmitis. Am J Ophthalmol 81:52, 1976
10. Michelson JB, Freedman SD, Boyden DG: Aspergillus endophthalmitis in a drug abuser. Ann Ophthalmol 14:1051, 1982
11. Ohno S, Kimura SJ, O'Connor GR et al: HLA antigens and uveitis. Br J Ophthalmol 61:62, 1977
12. Pettit TH, Olson RJ, Foos RY et al: Fungal endophthalmitis following intraocular lens implantation: A surgical epidemic. Arch Ophthalmol 98:1025, 1980
13. Peyman GA: Antibiotic administration in the treatment of bacterial endophthalmitis: II. Intravitreal injections. Surv Ophthalmol 21:332, 1977
14. Diamond JG, Kaplan HJ: Lensectomy and vitrectomy for complicated cataract secondary to uveitis. Arch Ophthalmol 96:1798, 1978
15. Diamond JG, Kaplan HJ: Uveitis: Effect of vitrectomy combined with lensectomy. Ophthalmology 86:1320, 1979
16. Belmont JB, Michelson JB: Vitrectomy in uveitis associated with ankylosing spondylitis. Am J Ophthalmol 94:300, 1982
17. Nobe JR, Kokoris N, Diddie KR et al: Lensectomy-vitrectomy in chronic uveitis. Retina 3:71, 1983
18. Fitzgerald CR: Pars plana vitrectomy for vitreous opacity secondary to presumed toxoplasmosis. Arch Ophthalmol 98:321, 1980
19. Belmont JB, Irvine AR, Benson WE et al: Vitrectomy in ocular toxocariasis. Arch Ophthalmol (in press)
20. Hagler WS, Pollard ZF, Jarrett WH et al: Results of surgery for ocular Toxocara canis. Ophthalmology 88:1081, 1981
21. Puig-Llano M, Irvine AR, Stone RD: Pupillary membrane excision and anterior vitrectomy in eyes after uveitis. Am J Ophthalmol 98:533, 1979
22. Michels RG, Ryan SJ: Results and complications of 100 consecutive cases of pars plana vitrectomy. Am J Ophthalmol 80:24, 1975
23. Peyman GA, Huamonte FU, Goldberg MF: Vitrectomy treatment of vitreous opacities. Trans Am Acad Ophthalmol Otolaryngol 81:394, 1976
24. Ballantyne AJ, Michaelson IC: Textbook of the Fundus of the Eye, 2nd ed. Baltimore, Williams & Wilkins, 1970

25. Hogan MJ, Zimmerman LE (eds): Ophthalmic Pathology: An Atlas and Textbook, 2nd ed. Philadelphia, WB Saunders, 1962
26. Yanoff M, Fine BS: Ocular Pathology. Hagerstown, Harper & Row, 1975
27. Saari KM, Solja J, Hakli J et al: Genetic background of acute anterior uveitis. Am J Ophthalmol 91:711, 1981
28. Hultsch E: Vitreous structure and ocular inflammation. In Silverstein AM, Michels RG, Green WR et al (eds): Immunology and Immunopathology of the Eye, pp 97–102. New York, Masson USA, 1979
29. Kampik A, Kenyon KR, Michels RG et al: Epiretinal and vitreous membranes: Comparative study of 56 cases. Arch Ophthalmol 99:1445, 1981
30. Gartner J: Elektronenmikroskopische Untersuchungen über Glaskoperrindenzellen und Zonulafasern. Z Zellförsch 66:737, 1965
31. Newsome DA, Linsenmayer TF, Trelstad RL: Vitreous body collagen: Evidence for a dual origin from the neural retina and hyalocytes. J Cell Biol 71:59, 1976
32. Gloor BP: Mitotic activity in the cortical vitreous cells (hyalocytes) after photocoagulation. Invest Ophthalmol 8:633, 1969
33. Intraocular Inflammation, Uveitis, and Ocular Tumors. Ophthalmology Basic and Clinical Science Course (Section 3). San Francisco, American Academy of Ophthalmology, 1981–1982
34. Smith RE, Nozik RM: Uveitis: A Clinical Approach. Baltimore, Williams & Wilkins, 1983
35. Wirostko E, Spalter HF: Lens induced uveitis. Arch Ophthalmol 78:1, 1967
36. Kanski J: Uveitic cataracts in children. Presented at the 11th Cambridge Ophthalmologic Symposium, St. John's College, Cambridge, England, September 10–11, 1981
37. Federman JL, Annesley WH Jr, Sarin LK et al: Vitrectomy and cystoid macular edema. Ophthalmology 87:622, 1980
38. Aaberg TM, Van Horn DL: Late complications of pars plana vitreous surgery. Ophthalmology 85:126, 1978
39. Peyman GA, Huamonte FU, Goldberg MF et al: Four hundred consecutive pars plana vitrectomies with the vitrophage. Arch Ophthalmol 96:45, 1978
40. Jaffe WE: Cataract Surgery and Its Complications, p 341. St Louis, CV Mosby, 1976
41. Pagrilli AMN, Belfort R, Abren MT et al: Ultrasonic fragmentation of cataract in uveitis. Retina 6:61–65, 1986

EIGHT

Endophthalmitis

The prompt recognition of endophthalmitis is of utmost importance. The earliest intervention should yield the greatest success in the true bacterial or fungal infection of the eye. In the majority of cases, bacterial endophthalmitis develops suddenly and progresses rapidly.[1] Suspicion is the most critical consideration in the presumptive diagnosis of endophthalmitis. All cases associated with penetrating ocular trauma or surgery need to be managed as likely candidates for an infection. Patients with endogenous endophthalmitis, usually those who are debilitated, immunosuppressed, or occult drug abusing patients, will be considered as a distinct situation within another setting. The classic signs and symptoms of a painful infected eye with hypopyon and vitreous inflammation do not always present themselves. The prudent suggestion for all suspected cases is the immediate performance of a vitreous tap, which is done best using a vitrectomy instrument. An anterior chamber paracentesis can be performed in the office. If one suspects endophthalmitis in a postoperative cataract with intra-ocular lens, where the posterior lens capsule is intact, a purely reactive inflammation may be present in the anterior segment of the eye. Paracentesis of the anterior segment may not yield either the cellular elements suggestive of infection or the evidence of bacteria or fungi essential to establish the diagnosis and to give the "green light" for either medical intervention or a pars plana vitrectomy.

The presence of an intact posterior lens capsule does not necessarily make the diagnosis of an endophthalmitis more difficult. The associated findings of conjunctival injection, hypopyon, decreased vision associated with cloudy or hazy vitreous in conjunction with the typical pain of endophthalmitis, strongly indicate the diagnosis. Prompt intervention before significant pain has developed will give one diagnostic anxiety, but the absolute absence of pain should make one question whether endophthalmitis or just reactive "uveitis" is occurring. Use of ultrasound in diagnosis can describe and pinpoint an inflammatory process versus a vitreous reaction, increasing vitreous opacities, or retinal choroidal thickening. Formation of anterior cyclic membrane can suggest early endophthalmitis. In the case of extracapsular cataract extraction, with or without intraocular lens placement, the development of strictly posterior inflammation would be very unlikely without any anterior segment involvement or full "spill-over," even with intact posterior capsule. Usually, however, the presence of an intact posterior capsule does appear to play a role in the amount of hypopyon that may or may not exist.

In order to distinguish an endophthalmitis from a sterile inflammatory reaction, the degree of inflammation and time delay in development of the inflammation are important. A postoperative sterile inflammatory reaction is usually seen within the first 24 to 36 hours; however, this should rarely be more than a minimal cell and flare development. The causes of sterile inflammation after cataract surgery include retained lenticular material, excessive vitreous manipulation, wound incarceration with iris, or reactive lenticular material encased in the vitreous gel. Vitreous hemorrhage and retinal detachment may occur in this setting and cause diagnostic confusion. These, however, are almost always painless conditions. It may occasionally follow an indolent course, associated with

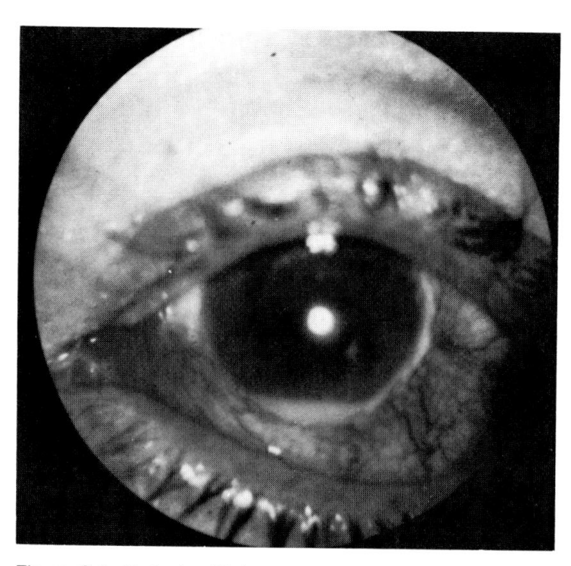

Figure 8-1. Patient with hospital-acquired s. epidermitis endophthalmitis whose organism proved to be resistant to all antibiotics.

cystoid macular edema and nonspecific iridocyclitis. It may also result from filtering blebs either in glaucoma surgery or from inadvertent wound leaks from cataract surgery. However, filter blebs are often implicated as the entry route for infectious endophthalmitis.[2-5] Should this situation continue or worsen 36 to 48 hours following a surgical intervention or penetrating injury, the likelihood of endophthalmitis is greater. While a number of supposed cases of endophthalmitis may prove sterile by culture, the initiating event is most likely to have been a *Staphylococcus epidermidis* or *S. aureus*.[4,6] It is noteworthy that, in recent years, the acquisition of hospital-acquired infections, which usually involve *S. epidermidis* and were once considered innocuous enough to be treated without vitrectomy and managed with topical subconjunctival and intravenous antibiotics alone, may now prove to be resistant to most of the drugs in our armamentarium (Fig. 8-1). These can present a particularly destructive problem for which mechanical vitrectomy and removal of the culture medium itself may be the only beneficial aspect of treatment (Fig. 8-2). The rule of finding a postsurgical inflammation greater than "normally expected" with one's surgical technique, should mandate entertaining a diagnosis of endophthalmitis and instituting appropriate management.

With a presumptive diagnosis of endophthalmitis, one is forced to follow one of two paths immediately. The first one is to perform a vitreous tap concomitant with intra-ocular antibiotics, steroids, and administration of intravenous antibiotic. This particular management regimen is directed toward those postcataract extraction infections diagnosed early. Generally, if the organism is of a *S.*

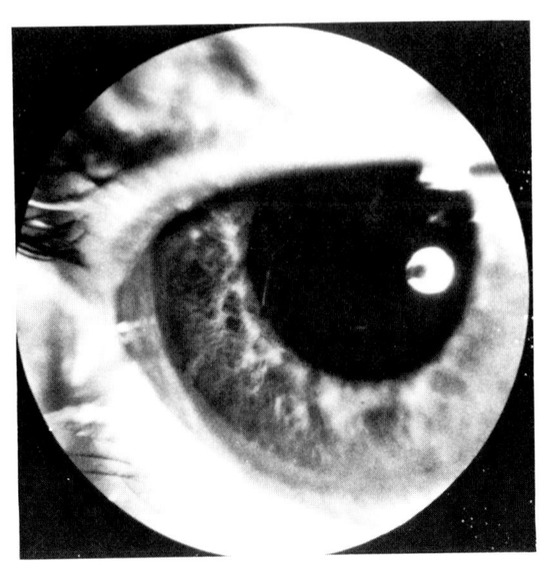

Figure 8-2. Patient with opaque media due to postoperative (cataract with posterior chamber lens implant) exogenous *Staphylococcus aureus* endophthalmitis.

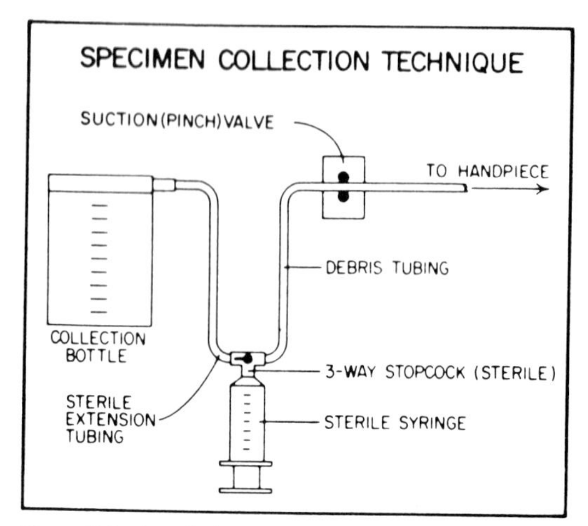

Figure 8-3. A technique for collecting uncontaminated specimens for culture during vitrectomy for endophthalmitis. (Courtesy Ronald E. Smith, MD, Newsletter v 3:2, 1978)

epidermidis, P acnes, or viridans staph variety, it will respond well to antibiotics, and full vitrectomy need not be entertained.[6–8] While some surgeons advocate needle aspiration of the vitreous in these types of endophthalmitis cases, either from the limbus or pars plana, most authorities have found that needle aspiration of the vitreous is cumbersome and occasionally dangerous. One must remember that vitreal-retinal band formation and organization of the vitreous may include many vitreal-retinal adhesions. Excessive manipulation of the vitreous in such a case may cause retinal tear formation which may be the inciting event of eventual proliferative vitreoretinopathy (PVR or MPP) which is, of course, catastrophic to the eye. These authors have found it difficult, if not impossible, to aspirate a typically turbid sample through a small 30- or 27-gauge needle, therefore necessitating use of larger needles, which may cause hazardous vitreous traction and unnecessary pulling on the retina with consequent retinal tear formation. We recommend using a 20-gauge vitrectomy instrument for all diagnostic vitrectomies in these cases. "One-incision" vitrectomy sampling is all that is necessary, using an anterior lavaging sleeve on the instrument itself. Careful manual suction and cutting are usually initiated and the syringe contents can then be sent for culture (see Fig. 8-3 for technique for collecting uncontaminated culture specimens). A central coring of the vitrectomy need not be undertaken in this situation unless one wants a more complete sample. In the case of routine infection, where an organism has not yet been cultured or identified at the time of vitreous biopsy, a dosage of 300 μg of gentamicin together with 2 mg of methacycline and 400 μg of dexamethasone may be instilled into the vitreous after a vitreous sampling has been performed.

Experimental and clinical evidence has now accumulated to support the combined use of intraocular antibiotics and therapeutic surgical vitrectomy.[9-21] Cottingham and Forster[22] have shown that eyes treated with both vitrectomy and intra-ocular gentamicin had significantly greater negative follow-up culture than those eyes tre ted with intra-ocular antibiotics alone. Removal of the core gel serves as an "incision and drainage" of the culture medium, removes the bulk of "sequestrae" infection from the eye, and converts the vitreous cavity into a permeable "sink" that allows more permeability of antibiotics, anti-inflammatory agents, and the natural flow of cells and humoral defenses.

When pars plana vitrectomy as a therapeutic regimen, over and above sampling of the vitreous for diagnostic purposes is entertained, one should direct one's thinking toward a central coring of the vitreous, as described previously. All patients with potential endophthalmitis associated with penetrating ocular trauma should be considered candidates for vitrectomy surgery, with careful consideration given to the antibiotics used in the infusion fluid. If a specific organism has not yet been cultured or its presence is suspected, 8 μg of gentamicin per ml, 9 μg of clindamycin per ml, and 10 μg of dexamethasone per ml may be added. This can be augmented by subconjunctival topical and systemic antibiotics for a period of four days. If the patient has been previously cultured in the office with an aqueous tap, one may wish to use organism-specific antibiotics, as indicated.

Whether or not intra-ocular lens implants should be removed in the course of pars plana vitrectomy for endophthalmitis is still controversial. In the past, removal of the intra-ocular lenses often resulted in significant bleeding and choroidal damage intra-operatively. An eye with significant inflammation and vascular congestion should be subjected to as little surgical manipulation as possible. As time has progressed, there seems to be less reason for removal of intra-ocular lenses in endophthalmitis. If visualization of the posterior segment is a problem, small corneal incisions can be made at the limbus; the vitrectomy instrument can be inserted into the anterior segment to remove fiber membranes that cover the anterior surface of the lens during vitrectomy and small capsulotomies can be made centrally in an intact posterior capsule. Insertion of the vitrectomy instrument through the pars plana incision then allows adequate removal of the vitreous with adequate visualization of the procedure. The lens is often of minimal hindrance in these circumstances. Diamond believes that the implant should be removed in cases of fungal endophthalmitis.[23] One should not perform extensive vitrectomy in the far periphery of the vitreous or posteriorly over the retina, which is often edematous and opaque, for all the reasons already outlined due to tugging on vitreal-retinal adhesions. Usually, at the termination of pars plana vitrectomy, subconjunctival antibiotics are given, usually 100 mg of methicillin, associated with topical gentamicin or tobramycin, or if a specific organism has been identified, antibiotics germane to that organism are used. Corticosteroids are usually favored in almost all cases of endophthalmitis. The dose of the intravitreal injection is 400 μg of dexamethasone or 10 μg per ml of

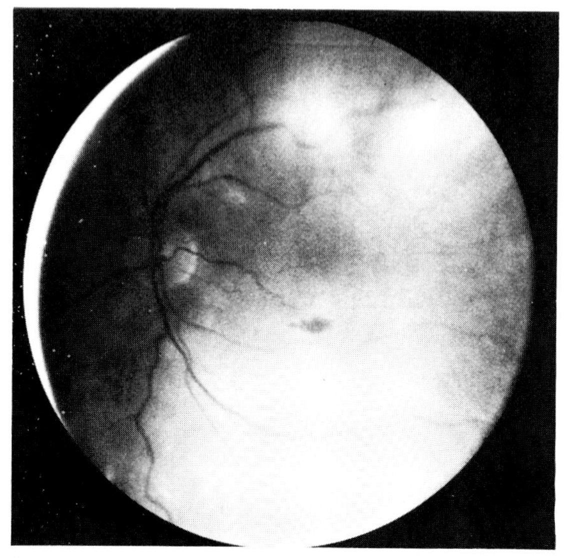

Figure 8-4. Immediate postvitrectomy view of the patient in Figure 8-2, whose retina demonstrates a small punctate hemorrhage inferior to the macula as well as profound retinal edema. The vision returned to 20/20.

the infusion fluid. The only contraindication to the use of steroids is that of a potential fungal endophthalmitis. If one suspects fungal endophthalmitis, these are usually avoided. A question has often arisen regarding the toxicity of intravitreal amphotericin in cases of fungal endophthalmitis. While the levels of toxicity are debated, a regimen of 10 to 5 μg of amphotericin B can be instilled into the vitreous at the conclusion of pars plana vitrectomy for fungal endophthalmitis.[24] Work by Peyman, Diamond, and others has shown that vitrectomy itself is often the curative factor in fungal endophthalmitis, over and above the intravenous and intravitreal instillation of amphotericin B, with or without miconazole or flucytosine. Patients with fungal endophthalmitis are often generally debilitated or sick and have other systemic causes of metastatic endophthalmitis. For these reasons, one may want to limit postoperative use of antifungal medications in patients with a metastatic process. In certain situations, they may already be on antifungal medication because of the metastatic process, for example, evolving from heart valve leaflets. In these situations, the pars plana vitrectomy is often a curative factor (Fig. 8-4).

Amphotericin B is a polyene active against all fungi that cause systemic infections. It is the most toxic of all antibiotics in clinical use today, and it should be given only every other day in doses not to exceed 1 mg/kg or a total of 3 grams. Although systemic mycotic infections are usually treated successfully, intra-ocular infections are rarely eradicated with systemically administered amphotericin B. The drug penetrates the vitreous poorly, even in inflamed eyes, and can be used only for the retinal lesions.[25] It is associated with many systemic side-effects including fever, chills, nausea, vomiting, renal failure, and bone marrow suppression.[28]

All the systemic side-effects can be alleviated by intravitreal injection of the medication.[28] Usually less than 10 μg can be injected intra-ocularly without retinal necrosis, but a dose of 1 μg has been reported as toxic in some retinas.[26–28] It is important that the needle be placed in the middle vitreous cavity with the bevel pointing anteriorly with a slow injection to prevent focal retinal necrosis. Stern and colleagues[25] reported a case of a 43-year-old heroin addict with *Candida albicans* endophthalmitis confirmed by culture; the patient was treated with a single intravitreal injection of amphotericin B. Seven weeks after treatment, the accidental death of the patient provided histopathologic evidence that the infection had cleared without toxic effects on the retina.

Flucytosine is a fluorinated pyrimidine readily absorbed from the gut with relatively few toxic effects and good penetration into the eye.[29] It is converted by enzymes in fungi to 5-fluorouracil, which is toxic to the metabolism of the fungus.[30] The emergence of fungal strains resistant to flucytosine makes it necessary to obtain culture results before beginning treatment with this drug alone.[30] Flucytosine and amphotericin B show some evidence of synergy,[29–31] although this combination may enhance the toxic effects of bone marrow suppression.[31]

Other antifungal agents have been tried. Intravenous nystatin has been used without success.[25] Miconazole and ketaconazole are imidazole derivatives with broad spectrum coverage and low toxicity. Like amphotericin B they alter the permeability of cell membranes, inhibit synthesis, and suppress proliferation and development of the pseudohyphae of *Candida albicans*.[29] Miconazole is poorly absorbed from the gut and must be administered intravenously, whereas ketaconazole is readily absorbed from the gastrointestinal tract. Both cause a transient rise in liver function tests, with hepatitis occurring as a rare complication. Ketaconazole alone may not reach therapeutic concentrations in the vitreous, but a combination of flucytosine and ketaconazole might be considered for the medical treatment of *Candida* endophthalmitis.[29]

The surgical treatment of *Candida* endophthalmitis includes vitreous biopsy and vitrectomy. Culture and microscopic examination of a sample of the vitreous fluid can be helpful when the diagnosis is in question, but the major emphasis in the surgical management of *Candida* endophthalmitis is on complete vitrectomy, with the removal of as much of the vitreous body as is feasible. This vitrectomy should be performed as soon as the diagnosis is suspected. The goals of pars plana vitrectomy are (1) confirmation of the clinical diagnosis with smears and cultures; (2) mechanical debulking of the vitreous body allowing better diffusion of medications in the vitreous cavity; and (3) excision of the vitreous gel to decrease or to prevent the formation of vitreoretinal traction bands.[30–32] When the vitreous cavity is involved, early vitrectomy is the key to successful treatment.[16,33,34]

The pars plana approach with bimanual intra-ocular instrumentation is preferred. Three incisions in the pars plana are needed. The first is for an intra-ocular infusion to replace fluid removed during the vitrectomy. The other two incisions are for endo-illumination and the cutting/sucking device. This bimanual approach allows better manipulation of the globe so that the instruments can be positioned where they are needed.

The several complications that can develop during vitrectomy are not necessarily unique to the treatment of fungal endophthalmitis. Subretinal infusion can occur if the infusion cannula has incompletely penetrated the vitreous cavity. This is avoided by checking to be certain that the cannula is in the middle vitreous cavity before irrigation is begun. Retinal tears can be created by vitrectomy. Special care should be taken during removal of membranes close to the surface of the retina over areas of inflammation, where the retina is frequently necrotic. Aggressive surgical manipulation should be avoided because retinal holes can be created by minimal traction over these areas. Also intra-ocular hemorrhage, lens opacities, and postoperative bacterial infections can develop.

The use of steroids in the treatment of *Candida* endophthalmitis is controversial. Steroids are contraindicated early in the course of the disease before antifungal agents have been started. Some surgeons prefer to inject steroids intra-ocularly at the same time as intra-ocular amphotericin to try to decrease the inflammatory response. Others prefer to wait 24 to 48 hours after injection of intra-ocular antifungal agents to begin steroid treatment. No definitive studies support either choice.

With evidence of systemic involvement or with positive blood cultures, systemic antifungal agents, with or without vitrectomy and intra-ocular amphotericin, should be the treatment of choice. However, without evidence of systemic involvement and without positive cultures, local treatment (i.e., vitrectomy with intra-ocular antifungal agents) is an alternative. Overall, vitrectomy combined with systemic and intra-ocular antifungal agents seems most efficacious in treating mycotic endophthalmitis.[29–32]

There has been no indication for repeated intravitreal antibiotic injections following pars plana vitrectomy. By the time a repeat injection would be considered, the effective results should already be noted in the eye, with a diminution of inflammation. This mandates administering adequate doses of intravitreal antibiotic at the conclusion of pars plana vitrectomy. Often the dose of 100 mg or less, as advocated by some specialists, is too little and usually impractical, resulting in less than bacterocidal levels within 24 hours. If one is considering repeating a regimen of intravitreal injection because of a continuing and threatening intra-ocular inflammation, it is preferable to perform repeat pars plana vitrectomy than to anticipate intra-ocular injections alone.

Recent data have associated an 80% incidence of retinal detachment with traumatic endophthalmitis. In these cases, all but two eyes have been lost due to proliferative vitreal retinopathy. These cases were associated with trauma alone and were not attributed to elective surgery. It is to be expected, therefore, that the incidence of retinal detachment in these patients is far greater and, indeed, an ensuing proliferative vitreal retinopathy is to be expected. Postcataract endophthalmitis, on the other hand, yields a rate of retinal detachment of 10% to 15%. These cases also generally tend to go into a state of proliferative vitreal retinopathy or massive periretinal proliferation, and the success rate in treatment of these patients is also abysmally low. This outcome is based on several factors, including the presence of large posterior tears and holes in the retina and the ability to peel epiretinal membranes, which themselves hold, pull, and cause traction on the retina, on its interior surface, while the same process is occurring beneath the retina and within its structure as well. The treatment of large or significant retinal detachment at the time of initial infection is usually successful. For cases such as this, aggressive management of pars plana vitrectomy is probably best withheld, because the surgery will result in unnecessary procedures to the eye. Once inflammation has subsided and the vitreous is organized sufficiently, peeling the vitreous membrane and removal of the organized vitreous and repair of a retinal detachment probably have the best chance for success, but success in such cases will tend to be minimal. Vision, the underlying goal, in all of these surgical and nonsurgical situations is going to be extremely poor in either case for patients who have sustained trauma and have large retinal detachments with concurrent infection.

References

1. Theodore FH: Bacterial endophthalmitis after cataract surgery. Int Ophthalmol Clin 5:59, 1965
2. Hattenhauer JM, Lipsich MP: Late endophthalmitis after filtering surgery. Am J Ophthalmol 72:1097, 1971
3. Yannuzzi LA, Theodore FH: Cryotherapy of post-cataract blebs. Am J Ophthalmol 76:217, 1973
4. Valenton MJ, Brubaker RF, Allen HF: Staphylococcus epidermidis (albus) endophthalmitis. Arch Ophthalmol 89:94, 1973
5. Abelson MB, Allansmith MR: Normal conjunctival wound edge flora of patients undergoing uncomplicated cataract extraction. Am J Ophthalmol 76:561, 1973
6. Forster RK: Etiology and diagnosis of bacterial postoperative endophthalmitis. Trans Am Acad Ophthalmol Otolaryngol (in press)
7. Forster RK: Endophthalmitis: Diagnostic cultures and visual results. Arch Ophthalmol 92:387, 1974
8. Forster RK, Zachary IG, Cottingham AJ, et al: Further observations on the diagnosis, cause, and treatment of endophthalmitis. Am J Ophthalmol 81:52, 1976

9. Maylath FR, Leopold JH: Study of experimental intraocular infection. Am J Ophthalmol 40:86, 1955
10. Zachary IG, Forster RK: Experimental intravitreal gentamicin. Am J Ophthalmol 82:604, 1976
11. Peyman GA, Herbst R: Treatment of bacterial endophthalmitis with intraocular injection of gentamicin dexamethasone: A case report. Arch Ophthalmol 91:416, 1974
12. Peyman GA, Vastine DW, Crouch ER et al: Clinical use of intravitreal antibiotics to treat bacterial endophthalmitis. Trans Am Acad Ophthalmol Otolaryngol 78:862, 1974
13. Peyman GA, May DR, Ericson ES et al: Intraocular injection of gentamicin: Toxic effects and clearance. Arch Ophthalmol 92:42, 1974
14. Kanski JJ: Treatment of suppurative intraocular infections. Br J Ophthalmol 54:316, 1970
15. May DR, Ericson ES, Peyman GA et al: Intraocular injection of gentamicin: Single injection therapy of experimental bacterial endophthalmitis. Arch Ophthalmol 91:487, 1974
16. Axelrod AJ, Peyman GA, Apple DJ: Toxicity of intravitreal injection of amphotericin B. Am J Ophthalmol 76:578, 1973
17. Peyman GA, Nelson P, Bennett TO: Intravitreal injection of kanamycin in experimental induced endophthalmitis. Can J Ophthalmol 9:322, 1974
18. Nelson P, Peyman GA, Bennett TO: BB-K8: A new aminoglycoside for intravitreal injection in bacterial endophthalmitis. Am J Ophthalmol 78:82, 1974
19. Bennett TO, Peyman GA: Use of tobramycin in eradicating experimental endophthalmitis. Albrecht von Graefes Arch Klin Ophthalmol 191:93, 1974
20. Schenk AG, Peyman GA: Lincomycin by direct intravitreal injection in the treatment of bacterial endophthalmitis. Albrecht von Graefes Arch Klin Ophthalmol 190:281, 1974
21. Pague JT, Peyman GA: Intravitreal clindamycin phosphate in the treatment of vitreous infection. Ophthalmic Surg 5:34, 1974
22. Cottingham AJ, Forster RK: Vitrectomy in endophthalmitis. Arch Ophthalmol 94:2078, 1976
23. Diamond JG: In Harrison TA, Diddie RR: Vitroretinal Newsletter 411, 1985
24. Axelrod AJ, Peyman GA: Intravitreal amphotericin B treatment of experimental fungal endophthalmitis. Am J Ophthalmol 76:584, 1973
25. Stern GA, Fetkenhour CL, O'Grady RB: Intravitreal amphotericin B treatment of Candida endophthalmitis. Arch Ophthalmol 95:89–93, 1977
26. Axelrod A, Peyman G, Apple D: Toxicity of intravitreal injection of amphotericin B. Am J Ophthalmol 76:578–583, 1973
27. Souri EN, Green WR: Intravitreal amphotericin B toxicity. Am J Ophthalmol 78:77–81, 1974
28. Wilmarch SS, May DR, Roth AM et al: Aspergillus endophthalmitis in an intravenous drug user. Ann Ophthalmol 15:470–476, 1983
29. Salmon JF, Partridge BM, Spalton DJ: Candida endophthalmitis in a heroin addict. A case report. Br J Ophthalmol 67:306–309, 1983
30. Snip RC, Michels RG: Pars plana vitrectomy in the management of endogenous candida endophthalmitis. Am J Ophthalmol 5:699–704, 1976

31. Doft BH, Clarkson JC, Rebell G et al: Endogenous aspergillus endophthalmitis in drug abusers. Arch Ophthalmol 98:859–862, 1980
32. Dishotsky NI, Loughman WD, Mogar RE et al: LSD and genetic damage. Science 172:431–439, 1971
33. Leopold IH, Apt L: Postoperative intraocular infections. Am J Ophthalmol 50:1225, 1960
34. Aguilar GL, Blumenkranz MS, Egbert PR et al: Candida endophthalmitis after intravenous drug abuse. Arch Ophthalmol 97:96–100, 1979

NINE

Drug Abuse and Ocular Disease

Drug abuse presents a major national health problem, affecting our children and disgruntled subcultures especially,[1-4] as well as whole industries in which recreational drug use is an accepted norm.[5] Five thousand people daily experiment with their first dose of cocaine; more than 25 million Americans are cocaine users.[6] A presidential adviser has been implicated in the use of cocaine.[7] Physicians are often the unwitting suppliers, as well as abusers, of drugs.

Drug abuse ushers in a host of new considerations in the medical management of patients with mysterious complaints and illnesses. A young person who has not undergone ocular surgery, and who presents with what appears to be a metastatic endophthalmitis should be suspected of intravenous drug use until proven otherwise. Patients who suffer metastatic endophthalmitis caused by either intravenous drug abuse or metastatic emboli due to drug treatment can have devastating damage done to their ocular structures before the etiology of this phenomenon is recognized and treated. Particulate matter may embolize to the eye, particularly in intravenous drug abuse patients who "cut" and dilute their intravenous substances with talc, cornstarch, and other particulates. These may embolize to the eye either in a shower or as a single focus of inflammation or infection.

Types of Abused Drugs

Opiates

The early use of opium seems to have been limited mostly to medical religious ritual. However, evidence exists that all of the major ancient civilizations had knowledge of the opiates, including the Sumerians at some time before 3000 B.C. By the 5th century B.C., Greek physicians recommended avoidance of opium. Homer's nepenthe was such a drug used to banish pain and sorrow. It may have been an extract of cannabis or a form of opium.

Arabs carried opium to Eastern Asia and the Indians, and Chinese incorporated it into their pharmacopaeia. When tobacco smoking began in the 1600s, the Chinese started to mix the substance with opium, and soon a drug problem was extant in all of China. At the same time, the Indians confined opium to medicinal and ritual use; therefore, it did not become a significant vehicle of abuse in India. By the middle of the 19th century, millions of Chinese men, but very few women, habitually smoked opium. Much of the opium used in China came from India, where it was imported by the British, eventuating in the opium wars of 1842 and 1858. The British triumphed, and China continued in its opium daze. Meanwhile, the West discovered morphine and invented the hypodermic syringe. Use of morphine during the Civil War produced a large wave of addicts in the United States. Morphine was first thought to be the answer to opium addiction. Then in 1898 a "cure" for morphinism was hailed. It was called heroin because it was thought to be the "heroic" cure.

Control of opium abuse began in 1875 with an act passed in San Francisco to suppress opium smoking. In 1914 the Harrison Narcotic Act imposed a tax on the importation and manufacture of opiates and cocaine, in effect outlawing these substances. Illegal use of opiates, especially heroin, continued at a chronic low level until the 1950s when a meteoric increase began in their use and abuse. The government responded by increasing narcotic penalties. The 1960s and early 1970s saw an epidemic rise in narcotic-related deaths as well as morbidity, especially in New York City.[8] In 1970 Congress passed a Comprehensive Drug Abuse Prevention and Control Act (Public Law 91-513). This act created a broad-based federal control of drugs that would be considered as "candidates of abuse." Unfortunately, this control has not stemmed a lucrative illicit drug market, which extends from Iran, Pakistan, and Afghanistan to France, Yugoslavia, Turkey, Germany, and Mexico, and finally wends its way surreptitiously into the United States.[9]

Depressants

Except for alcohol, the sedative-hypnotic drugs have had a shorter and less colorful history than narcotics. Bromine salts and the first medicinal sedatives came into use during the latter half of the 19th century and were followed by chloral hydrate and paraldehyde. Barbituric acid was synthesized in 1863, but the depressant activity of barbitol, and diethyl derivative, was not reported until 1902. Three years later, the Germans reported chronic barbiturate intoxication and withdrawal reactions. But not until 1950 did Isbell and co-workers[10] firmly establish the capability of barbituates to produce physical dependence. The discovery of other sedatives and hypnotics progressed with the growth of the drug industry. The later-arriving minor tranquilizers with pharmacologic qualities similar to the sedatives now account for a large share of the legally prescribed mind-altering drugs.

Stimulants

Besides the ubiquitous coffee, tea, and tobacco, stimulants commonly abused include the naturally occurring coca leaf, or its extract cocaine, and a synthetic amphetamine group. Coca was cultivated in the Inca empire as early as A.D. 1000. The Inca hierarchy employed coca in religious ceremonies to symbolize strength, endurance, and fertility. By the time the Spanish invaders arrived, its use was widespread and the Spaniards paid the Indians with slave labor and coca leaf. A Spanish physician who visited the Andes in 1555 wrote

> In certain valleys between the mountains grows a plant called coca, which the Indians value more than gold and silver. The mystery of this plant of plants is that those who chew its leaves never feel cold, hunger, or thirst.[11]

In 1858, Neiman isolated cocaine from the leaf and Western medicine began using it as a local anesthetic. Freud first extolled cocaine as a cure for morphine addiction, then changed his mind when one of his friends died from cocaine overuse. His close friend Kohler, a Viennese ophthalmologist, first instituted and later popularized its use as a local anesthetic for ophthalmic surgery. Even literary heroes indulged, such as Sir Arthur Conan Doyle's famous Sherlock Holmes, against the advice of his trusted friend, Dr. Watson. In the United States cocaine became an ingredient of some patent medicines and soft drinks; including one of America's most popular drinks, Coca-Cola. The Pure Food and Drug Laws, passed in 1906, and the Harrison Act banned this pattern, and cocaine use went underground. Since then the fashion for cocaine has varied. Its present popularity seems limited only by its high price.

Amphetamine, the first of the man-made stimulants, was synthesized in 1887 but not until 1928 did Alles describe its medical potential.[12] Other synthetic variants such as methamphetamine and methylphenidate soon followed. The amphetamines were used medicinally for treatment of nasal congestion, obesity, depression, and narcolepsy. Pediatricians and psychiatrists have used them (e.g., Ritalin) to subdue the so-called attention deficit disorder with or without hyperactivity in children. Users of amphetamines quickly noticed that euphoria may accompany the drugs' medical effect and abuse began. Now the drugs are on the

Federal Controlled Drug List, and medical authorities feel that synthetic stimulants have a very limited medical use except for those indications noted.

Hallucinogens

Hallucinogenic substances cover a wide spectrum from those naturally occurring in plants to the alphabet soup of synthetics and semisynthetics ("designer drugs") such as LSD, STP, PCP, MDA (D-lysergic acid diethylamide, 2,5-dimethoxy-4-methylamphetamine, phencyclidine, and methylene dioxyamphetamine). Mushrooms were used in prehistoric times and continue to be used in certain cultures. American Indians have used cactus-derived peyote for years, often as part of a religious ritual. Cannabis sativa can be loosely classed with the hallucinogens, and it can be obtained in a variety of forms from the hemp plant. Many historians cite its probable use by various ancient cultures. It was said to have been used around A.D. 1000 by a group of Moslem fanatics who were led by Hafan-Ibn-Al-Sabbah. Some etymologists derived the words *hashish* and *assassin* from the name *Hafan.* The argument continues as to whether the cannabis incited the fanatics to kill, or whether they merely used the drug as part of their lifestyle.

There is little interesting history germane to the more modern hallucinogens. LSD-25 or D-lysergic acid diethylamide was so named because it was found in 1938 during Dr. Hofmann's 25th experiment on derivatives from the ergot fungus. Dr. Hofmann, a Swiss chemist, 5 years later accidentally injected the drug and discovered its mind-altering properties. The hallucinogens remained in a world of esoterica until 1963 when Professors Leary and Alpert were dismissed from Harvard for conducting hallucinogenic experiments on their students. The attending publicity helped to add hallucinogens to the drug abusers' armamentarium.

Complications of Parenteral Drug Abuse

Methods of Administration

Drugs of abuse can be "snorted," smoked, injected into soft tissues ("skin popping"), or injected directly into a vein ("mainlining"). The most profound morbidity of drug abuse is associated with the intravenous injections of drugs. The drug culture is "indebted" to the treatment of schistosomiasis in Egypt in the 1930s for the introduction of the syringe as the ultimate vehicle for opiate abuse.[8] Interestingly, epidemics of falciparum malaria were the first by-products of this chronological advance, resulting from the communal use of needles without regard for absolute sterility. This necessitated the use of quinine as one of the elements to "cut" heroin in order to ameliorate the fever of malaria, which had been introduced into New York City and spread among the early heroin addicts of the 1930s.[8]

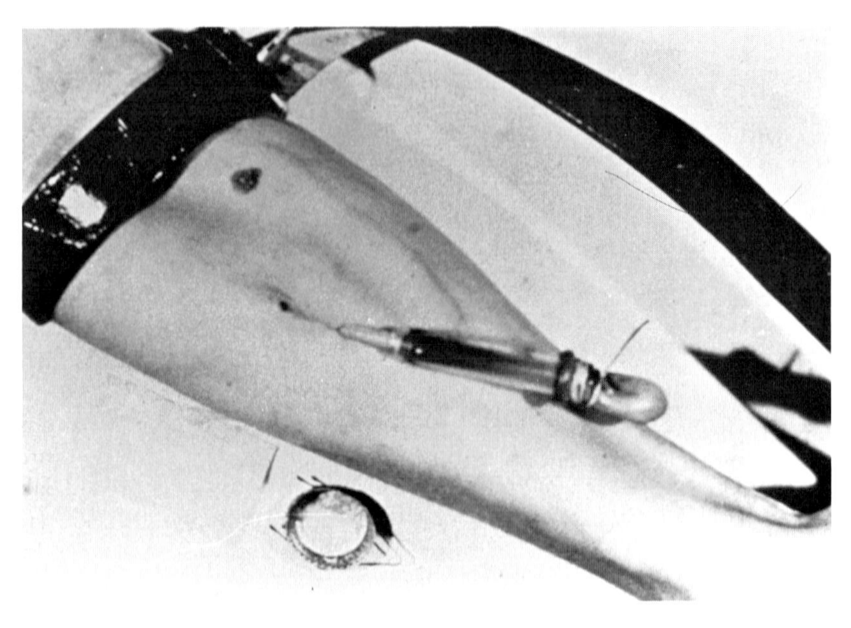

Figure 9-1. Typical crude, nonantiseptic, shared "needlecraft."

Currently, drugs are prepared for injection by dissolving a powder, tablet, or capsule in water heated in a small receptacle, frequently a bottle cap or spoon known as a "cooker." The solution is then drawn into a cylinder, syringe, or eyedropper known as "the works." A wisp of cotton may serve as a filter over the orifice to prevent injection of large particulate material undissolved in the heating process, but often this measure is unsatisfactory. The end of the needle is usually crudely sterilized over a match. When the needle is inserted into the blood vessel, blood is drawn back into the syringe and mixed with the drug-containing solution. Often, to verify that the contents were infused into the vessel, blood is drawn back into the cylinder and mixed with residual drug and then re-injected. "The works" are then passed to a companion who repeats the same procedure with the blood-contaminated needle and syringe or eyedropper (Fig. 9-1). The initial venous entry site is often the antecubital fossa (Fig. 9-2). These veins soon become sclerosed and the addict begins using the veins of the back of the hand or the lower extremities or other accessible vessels (Fig. 9-3). Attempts may be made to camouflage needle tracks with homemade tatoos (Fig. 9-4). Finally, the parenteral drug abuser will resort to skin popping, often into joint spaces and bursae, when he or she can no longer locate or inject into a subcutaneous vein. Skin-poppers frequently have circular, depressed scars on the thighs (Fig. 9-5).

Mechanism of Injury

The injection of abused drugs into the bloodstream of soft tissues may result in widespread tissue injury secondary to infection and to the introduction of drug

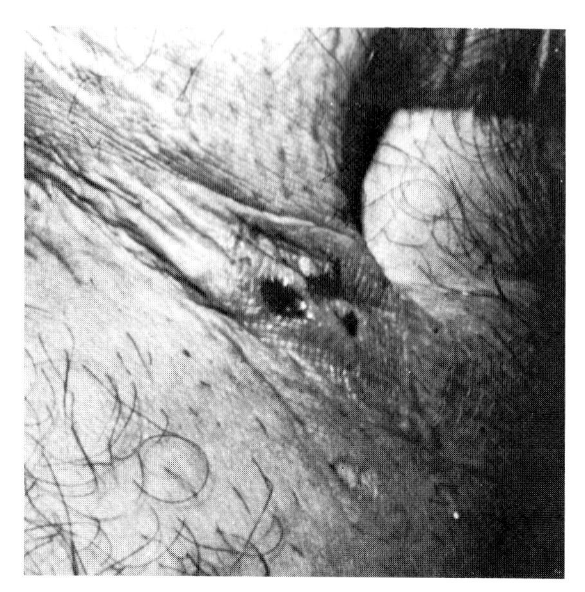

Figure 9-2. Characteristic linear, pigmented scars overlying fibrosed veins in the antecubital fossa may be the first external suggestion of intravenous drug abuse. (Courtesy Frank Raasch, MD)

and chemical contaminants (Fig. 9-6). Injection of foreign particulate material may overwhelm the immune system and lead to reduced immune responsiveness to infectious agents. The virulence of the human T lymphotropic virus (HIV) agent which causes AIDS in parenteral drug abusers is possibly related to the synergistic effect of antigenic overload from chronic exposure to chemical contamination with illicit drugs.

Drug and Chemical Injury

Drugs may cause injury through numerous reactions including toxic effects, allergic reactions, idiosyncrasies, and side-effects. A 37-year-old man developed an accelerated ventricular rhythm associated with the intravenous injection of cocaine.[13] Cocaine acts by enhancing cardiac automaticity through direct sympathetic stimulation, alterations at the peripheral nerve endings, and direct action on myocardial tissue. Respiratory collapse and death may occur rapidly after the intravenous injection of cocaine.[14] Cocaine snorting may cause severe damage to nasal tissues (Fig. 9-7). The Dallas County Medical Examiner's Office reported nine deaths in black male intravenous propylhexedrine drug abusers.[15] They suspected the mechanism of death to be a combination of cardiac arrhythmia with pulmonary hypertension and cor pulmonale.[16]

Necrotizing cerebral vasculitis, histologically similar to polyarteritis nodosa, was reported in an intravenous abuser of heroin, cocaine, and amphetamine.[17]

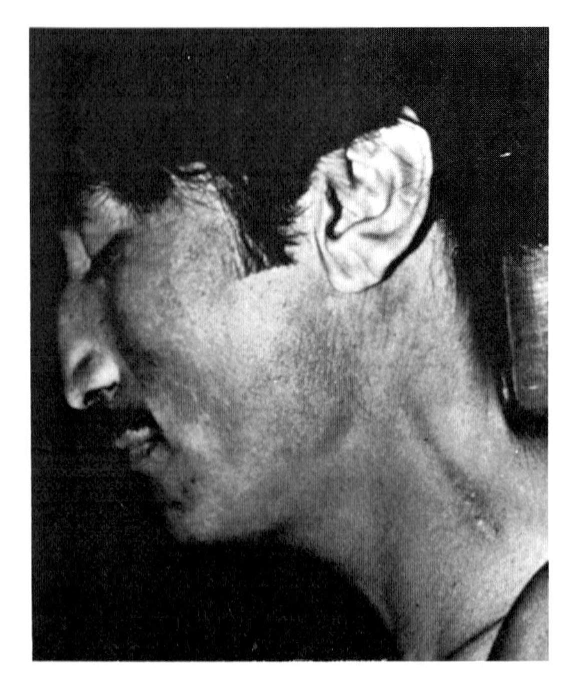

Figure 9-3. Addict injecting a mixture known as "blue velvet" scleroses the injected veins as shown in this patient's blue, fibrotic jugular vein.

The 22-year-old man presented with severe throbbing bilateral headaches and choked hyperemic discs before he became unresponsive from an acute hypertensive intracerebral and subarachnoid hemorrhage. Renal[18] and systemic[19] amyloidosis has been reported with chronic subcutaneous injections of pentatocine (Talwin). There are eight reported cases of accidental intra-arterial injection of oral drugs.[20] Complications include extensive tissue ischemia with loss of tissue. Two hard-core addicts with inaccessible veins developed an overwhelming, lethal, subcutaneous inflammatory reaction after "skin popping."[21]

Infectious Complications of Drug Abuse

The parenteral drug abuser is susceptible to a vast array of infectious agents including bacteria, viruses, fungi, and protozoa. The disregard for aseptic technique, contaminated illicit drugs and diluting substances, the sharing of injection paraphernalia by several people, and the direct infusion of organisms into the bloodstream or subcutaneous tissue are all responsible for these infectious complications.

Viral hepatitis is the most common infectious complication of addiction, usually the result of shared needles. Some 75%[22] to 98%[32] of parenteral drug abusers showed serologic evidence of hepatitis B virus infection, past or present,

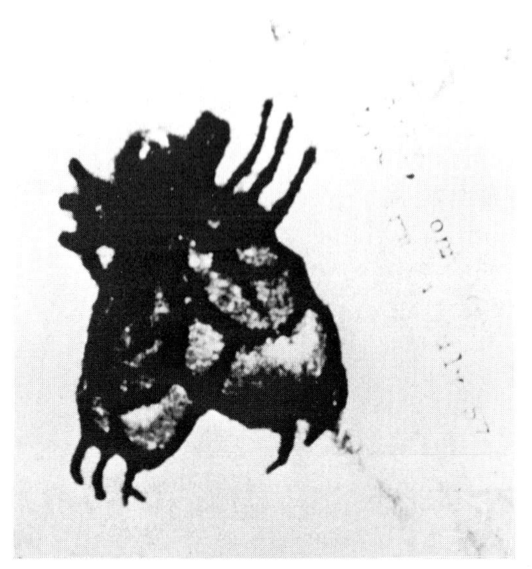

Figure 9-4. Frequently intravenous drug abusers will attempt to camouflage their needle tracks with homemade tattoos.

as compared with 13% of controls. Non-A, non-B viral hepatitis, defined by ALT (SGOT) elevation with negative HBV serology, occurred in 14.3% of drug addicts in a Sydney study,[22] 25% in a Swedish study,[23] and 20% to 25% in drug addicts in the United States.[24] Recently a hepatitis agent named delta (HDV) has been

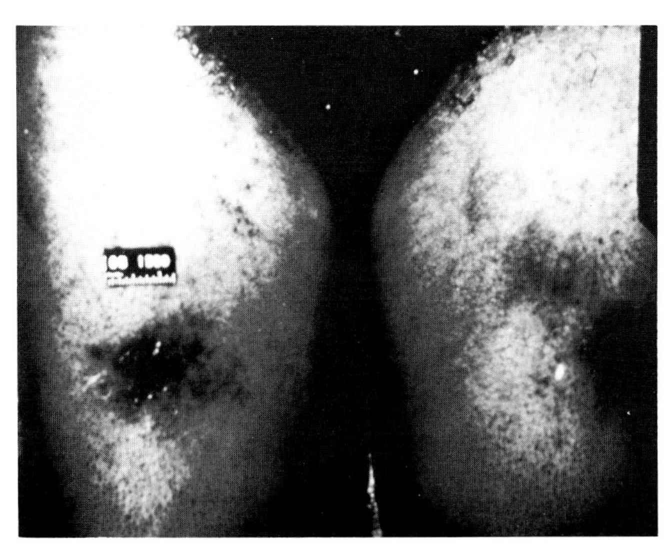

Figure 9-5. "Skin-poppers" frequently demonstrate characteristic circular depressed scars on the thighs.

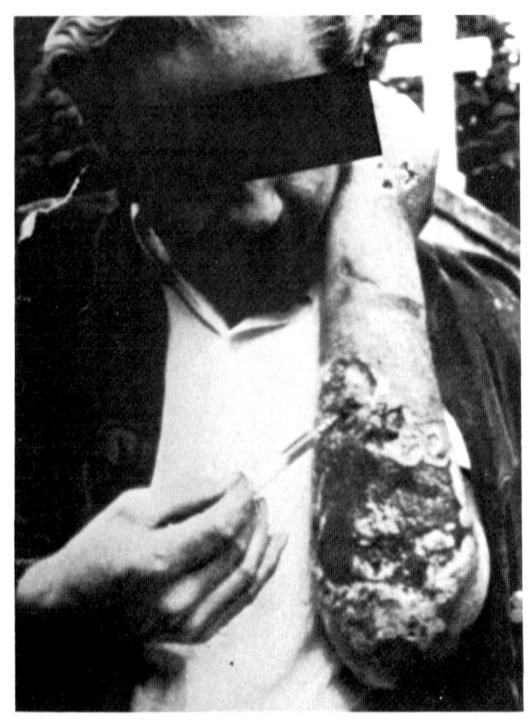

Figure 9-6. Prominent coalescing, depressed, and circular scars and ulcers covering unexposed areas on the trunk and extremities may indicate substance abuse. (Courtesy Frank Raasch, MD)

identified. It has an RNA genome and requires the hepatitis B virus to replicate HDV. In Anglo-Saxon countries, the HDV is virtually confined to parenteral drug addicts and their contacts.[25,26] In the United States there has been limited spread among homosexual men. The prevalence of serum delta antigen or anti-delta among addicts with HB_sAg-positive hepatitis was 64% (104/161) in Italy, 44% (8/18) in Denmark, 33% (11/33) in Switzerland, and 31% (15/49) in Ireland.[25]

Hepatitis B virus markers were detected in 43.6% (24/55) of drug addicts studied in the United States who were chronic HBV carriers.[29] An outbreak of delta hepatitis was reported in Worcester, Massachusetts,[28] in 1983. Of patients with acute hepatitis, 98% (49/50) had shared needles or had sexual contact with a parenteral drug addict. Fulminant hepatitis was a prominent feature of this outbreak and six patients died. As delta infection becomes more prevalent in the United States, it will most probably stimulate health professionals, homosexual men, and future intravenous drug abusers to obtain active immunity to the HBV with the Heptavax vaccine.[29]

Endocarditis, as well as endophthalmitis, in an otherwise healthy young person should suggest the possibility of drug addiction. Infective endocarditis is

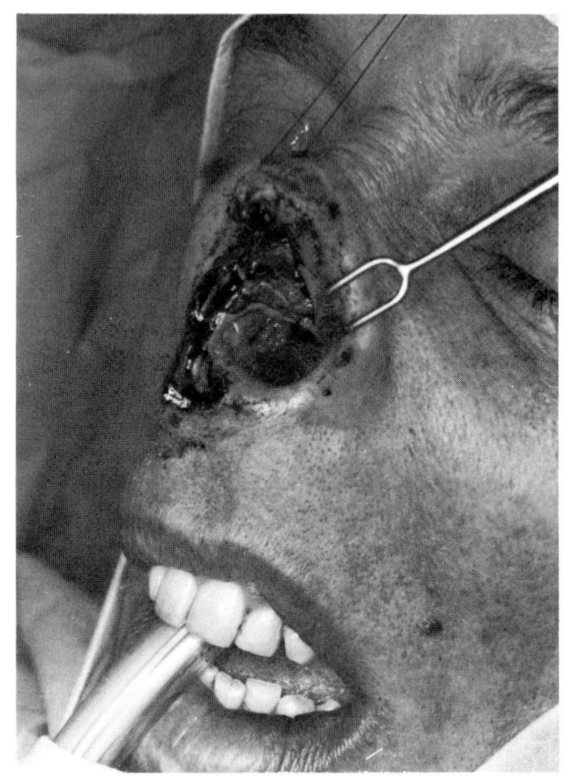

Figure 9-7. Erythema, ulceration, or perforation of the nasal septum reveals strong suggestive evidence of cocaine "snorting." (Courtesy Nicholas Schenck, MD)

now a frequent and well-recognized complication of parenteral drug addiction.[30] The aortic and mitral valves are the most frequently injured and also manifest the most prominent valve lesions. The most common bacteria isolated is still *S. aureus*.[32,33] Endocarditis due to *S. aureus* of identical phage type developed in two intravenous drug abusers who used the same paraphernalia for injections.[33] Other investigators have failed to recover a single isolate of *S. aureus* from street drug samples examined, although other organisms have been frequently cultured.[33] The spectrum of bacterial agents responsible is rapidly changing and now includes gram-negative rods, including *Pseudomonas*. A case of *Pseudomonas* endocarditis involving the tricuspid valve in a 20-year-old man was successfully treated with valve replacement after failure of medical therapy.[34] Mixed bacterial infection of cardiac valves has been reported in an amphetamine abuser.[35]

Fungal Diseases

Fungi, most commonly *Candida* species, are responsible for endocarditis with a resultant high mortality among intravenous drug users. Endocarditis due to fungal pathogens is a special problem in the addict population. More than 20% of cases of fungal endocarditis is associated with parenteral drug abuse. A 24-year-old heroin addict developed *Candida parapsilosis* infection of an artificial aortic valve.[36] The same organism was also isolated from all three syringes the patient had used for the injection of heroin. The patient cleaned his paraphernalia with a glucose-containing alcohol beverage that was thought to be a good culture medium for *Candida parapsilosis*.

Protozoan Illnesses

In the 1930s in New York City, 136 malaria-related deaths were recorded in heroin addicts.[8] A well-informed East Coast dealer added quinine to the heroin as the "cutting" agent to quell this frequent and fatal complication. With worldwide shortages of quinine, resurgence of drug-related transmission poses an ever-present problem. Servicemen returning from Southeast Asia with drug problems were incriminated as the source of malaria outbreaks in the late 1960s and early 1970s in the United States.

Neoplastic Complications

The cardiac surgery service at Roosevelt Hospital in New York City reported a statistically significant incidence of neoplastic disease in heroin addicts in the early 1970s.[37] The authors postulated a definite relationship between host resistance, addiction, and an imbalance that results in unusual infections and neoplastic disorders.

Acquired immune deficiency syndrome (AIDS) is the deadliest medical complication of parenteral drug abuse.[39,40] AIDS is defined for epidemiologic purposes to include previously healthy individuals between the ages of 28 days and 60 years who have no known history of an acquired or congenital immunosuppressive condition and who present with an illness at least moderately predictive of a defect in cellular immune function.[41] The high risk groups for AIDS include homosexual men (73%), intravenous drug abusers (17%), Haitians (4%), hemophiliacs (1%), and blood and blood products recipients (1%).[40] The use of intravenous drugs predisposes to AIDS through transmission of a retrovirus, HIV. Blood contaminated with the virus is passed from bisexual or homosexual drug abusers to addicts with whom paraphernalia is shared. Recently, HIV was isolated from the tears of an AIDS patient.[42] One in every six AIDS victims is a parenteral drug abuser. These patients are less likely than the homosexual patient to be white, well educated, or affluent.[43] Studies in New York City and other large cities in the eastern United States indicate that 80% of intravenous drug abusers have antibody to the HIV. The incubation period for AIDS can be as short as 6 weeks or as long as 5½ years. In the future, many of the presently asymptomatic addicted carriers will develop increasingly severe opportunistic infections that will bring them to medical attention.

When heterosexual transmission has occurred, it has primarily been from men, particularly male intravenous drug users. However, in Zaire, where the male to female ratio of AIDS cases has been reported to be 1.1:1, transmission from women to men many be more common than in the United States.[43] Of 42 African women in whom AIDS or AIDS-related complex (ARC) has been diagnosed, 24% were professional prostitutes. Interestingly, none of the African prostitutes had a history of parenteral or nonparenteral drug abuse.[43]

Toxic Manifestations on the Eye

Drugs and compounds used to dilute them can have toxic manifestations on the eye. Historically, quinine has been used as an antimalarial and an abortifacient, and recently has found more use to dilute heroin. A drug addict was reported[57] whose visual acuity improved initially when he discontinued heroin diluted with quinine and switched to methadone.

The typical history of quinine amblyopia begins with a patient who wakes up the day following drug use complaining of blindness. The fundus can appear normal early,[58] sometimes suggesting hysteria, although retinal edema with a cherry red spot of the macula, arterial attenuation with vessels visible only to the equator, hemorrhages, and severely constricted visual fields may be seen.[57–60] At first, the ERG is within normal limits but within a few days, it becomes abnormal.[57,58] With time, the visual fields contract and the optic discs become atrophic. Years later there may be residual visual field defects and persistent depression of the electroretinogram.[58]

Quinine exerts a direct toxic action on retinal ganglion cells,[58] but the role of ischemia based on retinal vascular insufficiency is also thought to be contributory.[57] Therapeutic attempts are designed to reverse vasoconstriction. Therapies and treatments that have been used include: oral, intravenous, retrobulbar, and subconjunctival vasodilators; digitalis; massage of the globe; paracentesis; bilateral stellate ganglion blocks; and carbon dioxide inhalation.[57,58]

Iris atrophy may be another complication of quinine abuse.[61] Segmental thinning of the pigment epithelium is seen with transmission defects best noted on retroillumination. Segmental atrophy of the iris sphincter muscle may also be present, presumably owing to an ischemic change in the anterior segment.

Ethchlorvynol (Placidyl), a nonbarbiturate hypnotic, is also implicated in toxic amblyopia.[62,63] Vision will return to normal with discontinuance of this drug.

Another substance of known abuse is toluene,[64,65] one of the volatile hydrocarbons sniffed for its euphoric effects. Adhesives, lacquer thinner, and spot removers contain toluene. Visual hallucinations are associated with its abuse. In one reported case,[64] the hallucinations continued for 4 months, and the patient was found to have diffusely abnormal electroencephalograms and visual evoked potentials. In another instance of toluene abuse[65] the patient demonstrated severe decrease in visual acuity and signs of severe cerebellar dysfunction, including gait ataxia, dysarthria, extremity ataxia, and horizontal nystagmus. Two months after cessation of the toluene abuse, vision returned to 20/30 bilaterally with minimal cerebellar dysfunction although visual evoked responses continued to be abnormal.

Fungal Endophthalmitis

Endophthalmitis is a catastrophe and an increasingly common ocular complication of intravenous drug abuse owing to the dissemination of a variety of organisms in the blood stream. Drugs intended for intravenous use are heated in spoons or bottle caps, drawn into a syringe or eye dropper through cotton or other homemade filters to remove the larger impurities, and then injected without cleaning the skin.[66] Frequently the same syringe is used by several persons. Endophthalmitis follows after these organisms enter the eye, or after septic emboli from infected heart valves lodge in the eye.

Candida Endophthalmitis

Candida has been reported in 12% of endocarditis cases among drug abusers, while only 12 cases of *Candida* endophthalmitis associated with intravenous drug abuse have been reported in the literature.[67–76] This surprisingly small number of cases suggests that this entity is under-reported and now too common for any further case reports in the literature.

Candida, a ubiquitous organism, can be cultured from the mouth, gastrointestinal tract, and female genital tract in 20% to 50% of the normal population.[77] *Candida* has been recovered from contaminated drugs, syringes, needles, spoons, and cotton used to filter drugs for injection.[77] Its presence is usually associated with abdominal surgery, immunocompromised or immunosuppressed hosts, widespread use of antibiotics, and intravenous drug abuse.[68,77] In the addict, *Candida* endophthalmitis can occur in the absence of systemic disease or immunodeficiencies.[68]

In the early stages of *Candida* endophthalmitis, the eye may be asymptomatic, especially if the lesions are located in the peripheral retina. Patients are usually symptomatic with complaints of blurred vision, ocular pain, or loss of visual acuity.[77] Unlike bacterial endophthalmitis, *Candida* endophthalmitis has an indolent course. The retinal or vitreous lesions can be diagnosed sometimes weeks after the last known history of intravenous drug use.

Unlike ocular candidiasis from a hematogenous source in an immunocompromised patient, with its high mortality rate and high systemic involvement,[77] only one case with systemic involvement has been reported in connection with ocular candidiasis in intravenous drug abusers. Horne and colleagues[70] reported a patient with unilateral *Candida* endophthalmitis with multiple subcutaneous abscesses of the scalp and beard; culture result identified *Candida albicans.*

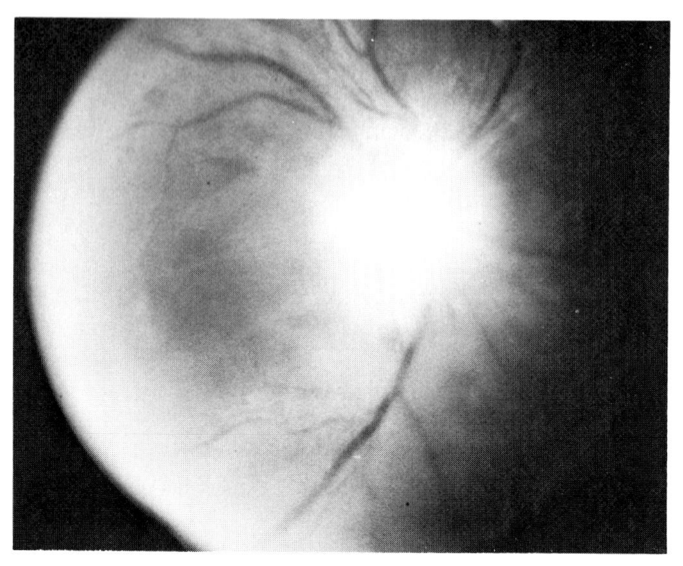

Figure 9-8. Typical *Candida* species puff balls in the vitreous due to metastatic fungal infection.

Candida endophthalmitis has many presentations, including nonspecific uveitis,[76,77] papillitis,[76,77] or nonspecific vitritis.[77] Most patients have an anterior chamber reaction and substantial vitreous involvement with cells and vitreous abscesses. The most common presentation of *Candida* from any source is a white, cotton-like, circumscribed exudate with a fluffy border located in the vitreous extending to the choroid and retina (Figs. 9-8, 9-9). Less frequent in drug addicts are the typical retinal lesions without vitreous involvement.[1]

The diagnosis of *Candida* endophthalmitis depends on a high degree of suspicion. A thorough history and suspicious visual examination of the patient should be undertaken, noting unusual skin lesions, nasal irregularities, tattoos, or other signs. Due to the variety of presentations, the diagnosis can be easily missed. If the typical retinal or vitreous signs are present in a patient suspected to have *Candida* endophthalmitis, a vitreous specimen must be obtained to make a definitive diagnosis.

Blood and urine cultures should be obtained to help rule out systemic candidiasis. *Candida* is a common culture contaminant, and the proper emphasis on reporting the organism can be overlooked even when typical colonies are grown. *Candida* can be difficult to grow on culture media, and multiple samples must be obtained to increase the chances of recovering the organism. The eye may be the only obvious organ involved in drug abuse, and systemic cultures may be consistently negative.

The diagnosis must be confirmed surgically. Anterior chamber paracentesis has yielded *Candida* organisms on culture, but usually a vitrectomy specimen is necessary. The vitreous aspirate should be filtered through a Millipore filter and

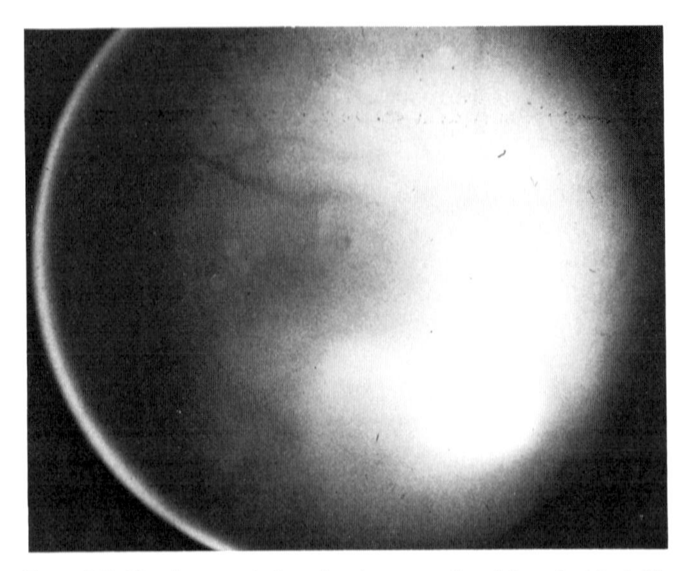

Figure 9-9. Classic presentation of endogenous *Candida* endophthalmitis in a drug abuser who demonstrates prominent vitreous fluff balls amid diffuse vitreous cellularity and haze.

concentrated since *Candida* can be difficult to grow from the vitreous. Cultures should include at least blood agar, chocolate agar, Sabouraud's agar, and thioglycolate broth. Slides should be prepared for Gram's stain, Giemsa stain, and KOH prep for microscopic study (Fig. 9-10).

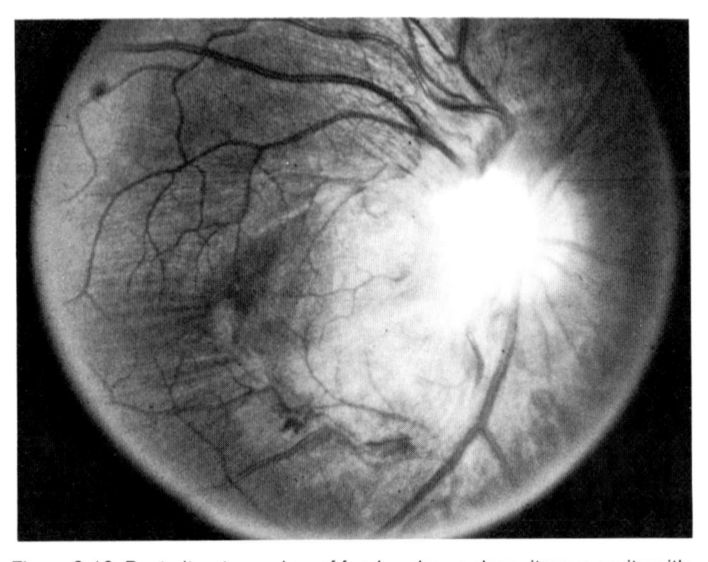

Figure 9-10. Post-vitrectomy view of fundus shows clear vitreous cavity with cellophane wrinkling changes in the internal limiting membrane of the retina.

Histopathologically a granulomatous and acute suppurative necrotic reaction is present.[77] Most eyes have multiple lesions, usually located in the posterior pole and less than 1 mm in diameter. The lesions are slightly elevated and have a smooth surface. Underlying depigmentation leads to transillumination defects. The lesions begin in the inner aspect of the choroid, destroying the retinal pigment epithelium, and extending into the overlying retina. Leukocytes are present in the adjacent vitreous.[77] Frequently only a small number of *Candida* organisms are found in the vitreous cavity, sequestered within white blood cell infiltrates.[1]

The prognosis for vision depends on how early the patient presents and treatment is begun. Four of twelve eyes treated early had return of vision to 20/40 or better.[67-70] The other eight eyes treated later in the course of the infection had final visual acuities ranging from 20/200 to no light perception. Generally a poor outcome can be expected once vitreous involvement has become established.[75] The overall prognosis can be related to a delay in presentation by drug abusers. Also, patients with suspicious symptoms may not be asked about or admit to intravenous drug use. The diagnosis may not be considered because many patients respond initially to steroids prescribed for uveitis.[69,75] Also, evidence of systemic candidiasis may be absent, and the results of a thorough laboratory evaluation may be negative.

Aspergillus Endophthalmitis

Aspergillus endophthalmitis is the second most common mycotic endophthalmitis found in intravenous drug users. *Aspergillus* is a ubiquitous organism in the environment and can be cultured from the normal human upper respiratory tract, as well as from dust and air. It has a uniform 3 to 4 μM hyphae with septae and characteristic 45-degree dichotomous branching (Fig. 9-11). It will stain with hematoxylin and eosin, but is seen better with methenamine-silver or other special fungal stains.[38]

Six cases have been reported in the literature: four cases of *Aspergillus flavus*, one case of *Aspergillus fumigatus*, and one nonspecific *Aspergillus* species.[28,68,75,78,79] The initial visual complaints were decreased visual acuity, pain, and conjunctival injection of the involved eye. All cases were unilateral. Anterior chamber reaction, keratic precipitates, conjunctival injection, and hyphema were described, along with vitritis and a white vitreal mass (Fig. 9-12). Retinal detachment was described in five of the six cases. Two eyes were enucleated[75,80] and one became phthisical.[79] In three eyes the vision returned to 20/200 or better.[68,78,79] In only one case were there specific details related to systemic involvement;[78] that patient was found to have *Aspergillus* osteomyelitis of a rib (Fig. 9-13). Two additional unusual cases of mycotic infection in intravenous drug users have been reported. Stenson and colleagues[81] described a bilateral necrotizing scleritis due to *Aspergillus oryzae* in a 40-year-old woman who used intravenous cocaine and heroin. *Aspergillus oryzae* is one of the least common *Aspergillus* isolates in man,

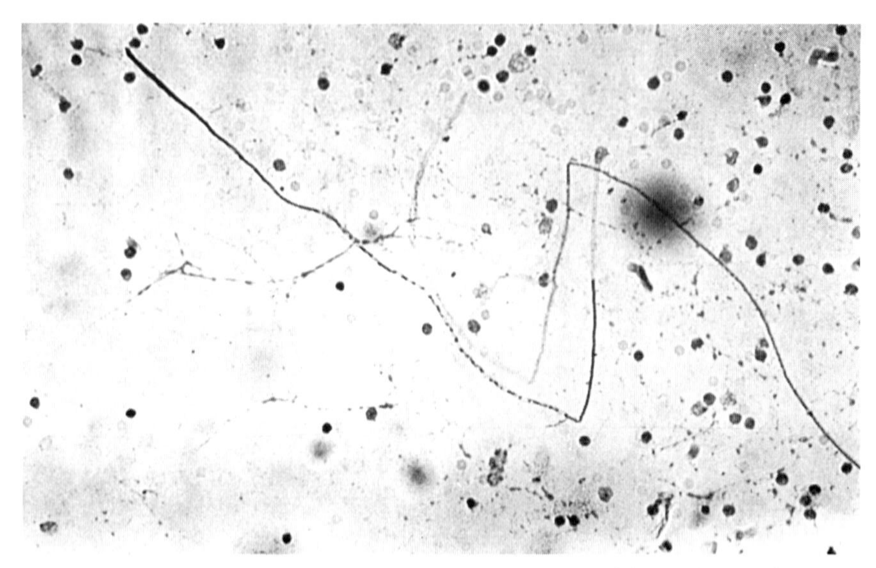

Figure 9-11. Vitrectomy specimen discloses the septate hyphae of *Aspergillus* species.

and this was the first and only reported case of the ocular involvement of this fungus in a human. The second case involved a 42-year-old woman with an initial unilateral endophthalmitis from which *Aspergillus flavus* and *Torulopsis glabrata* were cultured. After treatment with topical natamycin and flucytosine, the endophthalmitis recurred and a helminthosporium species was isolated. This pa-

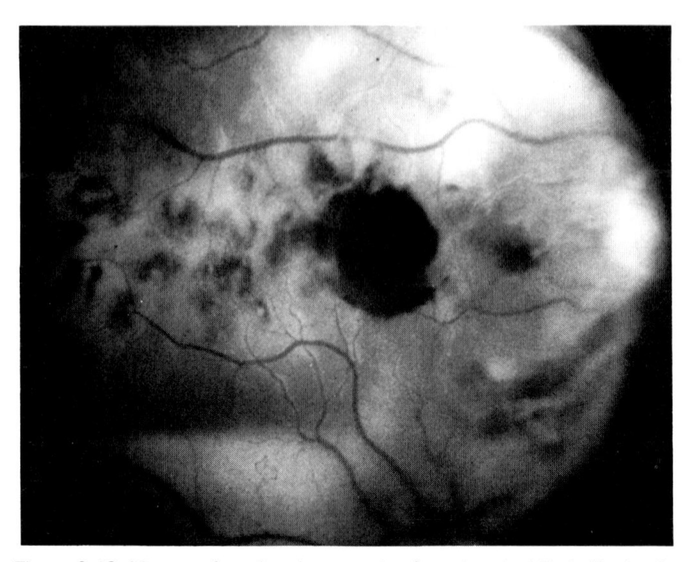

Figure 9-12. More profound and aggressive fungal endophthalmitis due to *Aspergillus* species demonstrating a meniscus of exudate under the retina.

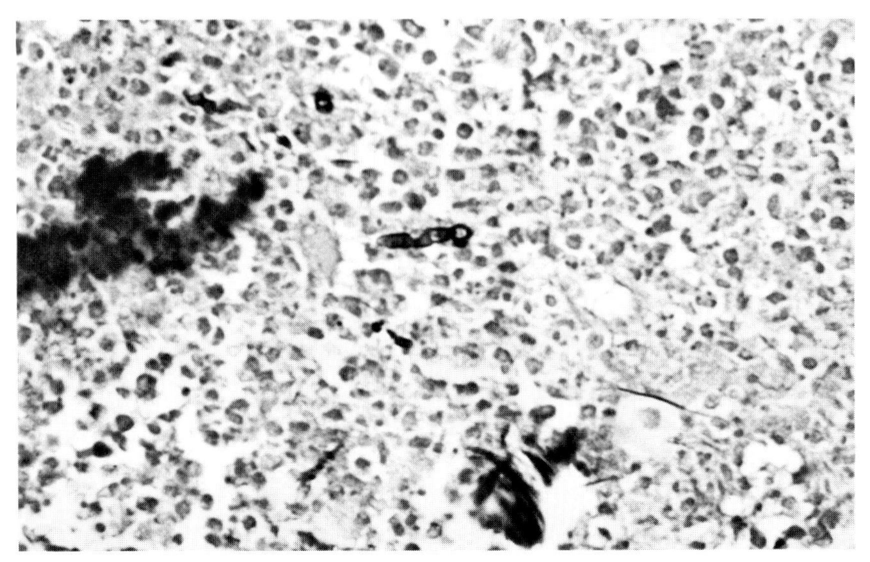

Figure 9-13. Portion of bone from a drug-abusing patient who suffered not only *Aspergillus* endophthalmitis but simultaneously developed *Aspergillus* osteomyelitis, which proved equally difficult to treat with amphotericin B and flucytosine therapy.

tient's husband, also an intravenous drug abuser, developed a *Candida* endophthalmitis 1½ years later.

The treatment of other less common kinds of mycotic endophthalmitis in drug addicts is the same as for *Candida* endophthalmitis, the prototype of this group of infections. From the literature, it appears that treatment of other mycotic infections has had less satisfactory results, possibly because of a lack of experience with these unusual organisms.

Bacterial Endophthalmitis

Bacterial endophthalmitis as an ocular manifestation of drug abuse is much less commonly reported than mycotic endophthalmitis. Most reported cases have been in association with acute bacterial endocarditis secondary to intravenous drug use.[82,83]

Acute bacterial endocarditis has been estimated to be present in 8% of the heroin addicts in Washington, D.C.[84] It is usually caused by an extremely virulent organism of high pathogenicity. In the above study, *Staphylococcus* species were the predominant organisms accounting for 75% of cases. *Streptococcus* species were the next most common, accounting for 14% of cases. Only one of 50 cases studied was found to be caused by *Candida*. Because of the virulence of the infecting organisms, metastatic abscesses can develop in other body tissues, but serious sequelae from septic embolization to the eye in endocarditis are rare.[85]

Patients with bacterial endophthalmitis present with symptoms of pain, redness, lid swelling, and decreased vision. Unlike the more indolent course in mycotic endophthalmitis, bacterial endophthalmitis can have an explosive onset with rapid progression.

Signs usually manifest in the first 24 to 48 hours after onset (Fig. 9-14). An intense anterior and posterior inflammatory reaction is usually present. Vision is decreased. Other reported ocular signs of bacterial endocarditis leading to endophthalmitis include cotton-wool spots and white, centered, flame-shaped hemorrhages, so-called Roth spots.[85] Banks and co-workers[84] reported three cases of unilateral, purulent panophthalmitis in 28 heroin addicts with infective endocarditis. Burns[86] reported a patient who had developed bilateral endophthalmitis associated with acute bacterial endocarditis of unspecified etiology.

The diagnosis of bacterial endophthalmitis in drug abusers again depends on a high degree of suspicion in the clinician. The diagnosis should be confirmed surgically. Many of the systemic antibiotics used in the treatment of endophthalmitis have side-effects that warrant a culture-proven diagnosis prior to prolonged therapy with these agents.

Treatment begins with pars plana vitrectomy, with vitreous specimens for culture and sensitivity studies and for histopathology (Fig. 9-15). The vitreous should be cultured on the same media used for mycotic endophthalmitis culture (blood agar, chocolate agar, Sabouraud's agar, and thioglycolate broth) and the same slides (Gram's and Giemsa stain, and KOH) prepared for microscopic study.

As in mycotic endophthalmitis, intra-ocular and systemic antibiotics are utilized in the treatment of intra-ocular infections. We use broad spectrum

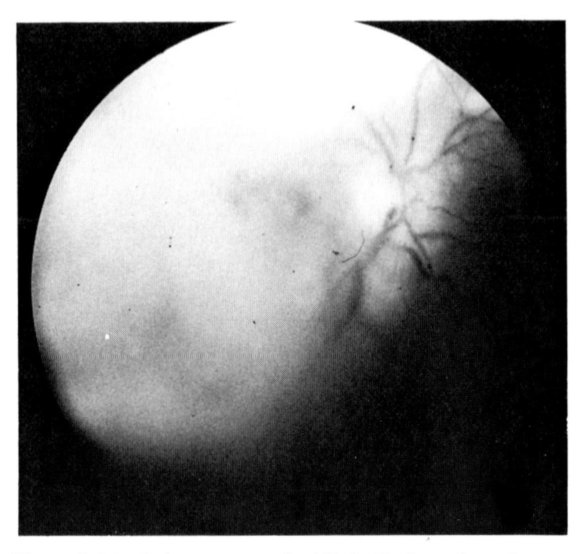

Figure 9-14. Endogenous endophthalmitis in a drug abuser. Only 3 days after injecting cocaine, his vitreous filled with dense white exudate.

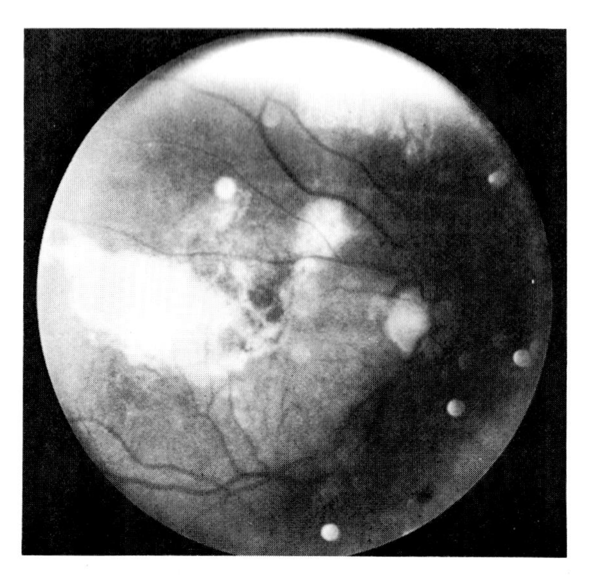

Figure 9-15. Postoperative view of fundus demonstrates fibrous scarring of the retina with visual return to 20/70, after intensive intravenous therapy with amphotericin B and flucytosine.

intra-ocular coverage until we have culture-proven results with antibiotic sensitivities. We use gentamicin (300 μg) and cefazolin (2.2 mg) intra-ocularly, taking the same precautions as with the treatment of mycotic endophthalmitis, that is, the needle is placed in the middle vitreous cavity with the bevel pointing anteriorly and the drugs are injected slowly. Gentamicin and cefazolin are also given subconjunctivally and systemically. The patient must also have a complete physical examination with blood cultures and also cardiology and infectious disease consultations to rule out endocarditis.

Bacillus cereus is usually nonpathogenic to man, but six cases of *Bacillus cereus* endophthalmitis have been reported in intravenous drug abusers.[87-89] This organism is particularly devastating to the eye, because of its numerous tissue toxins, including lecithinase.[89] *Bacillus cereus* is the most common organism cultured from street-acquired heroin and injection paraphernalia.[87]

Other septic retinal complications of intravenous drug abuse include a septic submacular choroidal embolus associated with heroin and phenmetrazine (Preludin) abuse, reported by Limage and Goldberg.[90] The patient did not have endocarditis and all blood cultures showed no growth. The macula became scarred, and final visual acuity was 20/200. Jarrett and Christy[85] reported the formation of a retinal hole in the macula after presumed septic embolus from bacterial endocarditis. Also Eichner and Aebi[91] reported on seven prisoners who injected a homemade alcoholic beverage and developed septic retinitis.

Acquired Immune Deficiency Syndrome

Another disorder associated with intravenous drug abuse is the acquired immune deficiency syndrome (AIDS).[92–100] AIDS is a severe disorder in which depression of the patient's cellular immune system results in subsequent development of multiple opportunistic infections, unusual neoplasms, and inability to mount a delayed hypersensitivity response. There is a profound defect in cell-mediated immunity, with lymphopenia, and a selective defect in the ratio of helper to suppressor T lymphocytes.[92–100] This syndrome is most commonly seen in homosexual men between 20 and 50 years of age and is also associated with Haitians, blood product recipients, intravenous drug abusers, and heterosexual contacts of individuals with AIDS.

The major ocular manifestations of this disease are cytomegalovirus (CMV) retinitis, cotton-wool spots, and conjunctival Kaposi's sarcoma.[97,99] Cytomegalovirus retinitis, which is a major cause of visual loss in AIDS, appears as a late finding, resulting from hematogenous dissemination of CMV to the retina. Cotton-wool spots do not appear to be due to infectious agents. Their presence implies microvascular alterations in AIDS.[97,98]

Other ocular manifestations of AIDS include cranial nerve paralysis, choroidal *Mycobacterium avium*, Mycobacterium *intracellularis*, *Cryptococcus*, and toxoplasmosis retinitis.[95–97,99,100] Ocular motility disorders in patients with AIDS should suggest an infectious or neoplastic meningitis. In general, motility disorders are seen later in the course of the disease.[98]

At the present time, the retrovirus as the etiology of AIDS is the hypothesis with the most convincing evidence, although other viruses including herpes, CMV, Epstein-Barr, hepatitis, adenovirus, and African swine fever virus have been suggested as possibilities.[101] A possible role for inhalant drugs (amyl, butyl, or isobutyl nitrite) in an immunosuppressive role as a cofactor in the establishment or outcome of the disease has not been ruled out. There appears to be a risk for blood-borne transmission of the disease, which may account for the incidence of AIDS among hemophiliacs,[101] while the sharing of needles may account for the disease among intravenous drug abusers. At the present time there is no specific treatment for the underlying immunodeficiency, only the management of opportunistic infections or tumors that develop as sequelae (see Chap. 10).[101]

Talc Retinopathy

In 1972 Atlee first described talc retinopathy in 17 drug addicts who had injected methylphenidate hydrochloride (Ritalin) intravenously. Since then talc retinopathy has been reported with the abuse of intravenous methylphenidate hydrochloride (Ritalin),[83,102–104] intravenous heroin,[105] intravenous methadone,[106] intravenous codeine,[107] intravenous meperidine (Demerol),[108] and intravenous pentazocine (Talwin).[109] Methylphenidate tablets contain talc (magnesium silicate) and cornstarch as fillers and binders, and are meant for oral use. However, the abuser prepares a suspension for injection by dissolving the crushed tablets in boiling water. The turbid solution may be passed through cotton or other home-made filters to remove the larger impurities. The filtrate is then injected intravenously, subcutaneously, or intramuscularly. The particles embolize to the lungs, causing pulmonary hypertension, and cor pulmonale. After some time, collateral vessels develop around the normal pulmonary circulation allowing particles to pass into the systemic circulation.[83,104,110]

In the eye, most of these particles settle out in the posterior retinal and choroidal circulation due to the dense capillary network and the greater blood flow to this area.[83] Ophthalmoscopically they appear as tiny glistening yellow crystals concentrated along the small arterioles of the perifoveal arcade in the posterior pole.[110] Also, micro-aneurysmal dots, enlarged arterial segments, venous loops, and retinal granuloma may be seen.[111] The talc emboli are found in the capillaries of the nerve fiber layer, internuclear layer, and choriocapillaris. No evidence of occluded vessels or granulomatous reaction around the vessels was found by Murphy and co-workers.[106]

Talc retinopathy develops only when this type of drug abuse is prolonged. Murphy and colleagues found it in 9 out of 17 intravenous methadone abusers. Emboli were present in all of the patients who had injected more than 12,000 pills but in none who had injected fewer than 9,000 pills. Schatz and Drake[104] found that all patients with talc emboli had used intravenous methylphenidate for more than 1 year, and most had used intravenous drugs for more than 3 years. These authors were unable to produce ophthalmoscopically visible talc particles in the monkey fundus by injecting intravenous methylphenidate three to four times per week for 3 months. Jampol and colleagues[111] did produce talc emboli by injecting Rhesus monkeys with talc intravenously twice a week for 3.5 to 10 months. In this work, the talc was seen in the fine perifoveal capillaries within one month. Friburg and co-workers[103] were the first to describe bilateral visual loss and irreversible macular ischemia from talc emboli in an intravenous methylphenidate abuser.

In patients with talc retinopathy, fluorescein angiography reveals precapillary arterial occlusions, capillary nonperfusion, an abnormal foveal avascular zone, and retinal vascular leakage.[104,109,111] Electroretinograms are usually normal even in patients with advanced talc retinopathy.[111] In addition, these patients develop large areas of capillary nonperfusion in the peripheral retina with resultant ischemia that leads to peripheral vasoproliferation.[83,110,111] Neovascularization develops at the border between the perfused and nonperfused retina.[109] This proliferation fits the Goldberg classification of proliferative sickle cell retinopathy. Such patients develop all the peripheral signs of sickle cell retinopathy except for the black sunbursts and salmon patches.[104] This proliferation can lead to disc neovascularization,[102] vitreous hemorrhage,[112] traction retinal detachment, or rhegmatogenous retinal detachment.[111] Talc retinopathy can be used as a model of sickle cell retinopathy.[110]

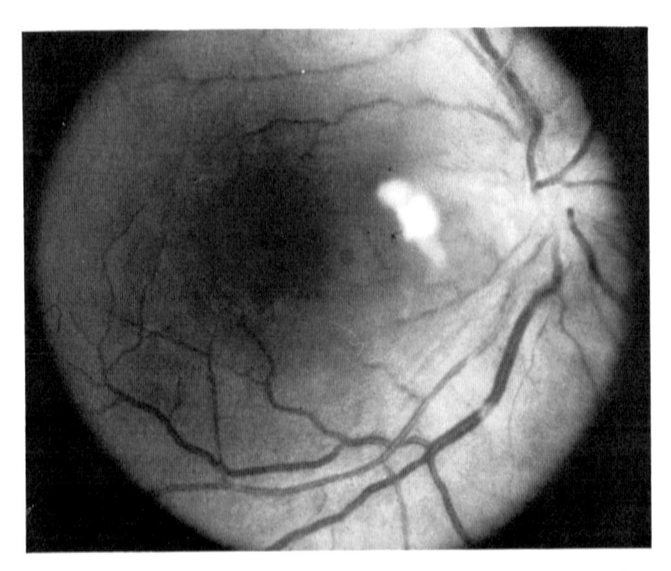

Figure 9-16. Fundus photograph discloses a large, solitary particulate talc embolism lodged in the papillomacular bundle of this intravenous cocaine abuser.

Keane[58] described one further cause of talc retinopathy. His patient was a 37-year-old chronic drug abuser who inadvertently injected the contents of codeine tablets into his left carotid artery, resulting in acute, left cerebral hemisphere stroke, and multiple branch artery embolic occlusions. Usually intravenous drug abusers who inject into the arterial circulation do so in the arteries of the extremities resulting in ischemic damage to the hands and feet.

The differential diagnosis of talc retinopathy should include macular drusen, fundus albipunctatus, retinopathy of Bietti's crystalline corneal dystrophy, cystinosis, and oxalosis.

Psychological Manifestations

Besides pharmacologic and infective manifestations of drug abuse, psychologic effects of drugs can also lead to ophthalmic manifestations. Solar maculopathy or foveal macular retinitis is one such entity. It has been reported that patients using hallucinogenic drugs experience more vivid "trips" by focusing their attention on bright lights such as the sun.[113] Several reports of solar maculopathy related to this habit have been described.[113-115] The mydriatic and cycloplegic effects of hallucinogenic drugs, particularly LSD, make their users susceptible to this disorder. Usually patients complain the next day of blurred vision, metamorphopsia, and central scotomas. Findings include decreased visual acuity of 20/40 to count fingers. The macula is described as "honeycombed" with a "hole-like" foveal lesion (Fig. 9-16).[115] There is usually a normal fluorescein angiogram throughout all stages of the disease, but occasionally early choroidal fluorescence is seen in the late stages of solar maculopathy.[113] Vision usually improves from the initial presentation but severe visual loss has been reported.[113] There is some question as to whether steroids help in the treatment of this condition.[114]

A recent report by Sadun and co-workers[115] has defined a number of factors that affect the extent of a solar thermal burn on the retina. These include (1) the sun's altitude (greater than 30 degrees from the horizon); (2) clear climatic conditions; (3) emmetropic refractive error; (4) clear optical media; and (5) use of analgesics to reduce sensitivity to the sunlight burn. In both of the cases presented, 30 to 60 seconds of staring at the sun sufficed to produce a thermal burn of the retina.

There have also been several reports of self-enucleation by drug abusers.[116,117] In both references the patients were preoccupied with religious thoughts and referred to Matthew 5:22: "and if thy right eye offend thee, and if thy right hand offend thee, cut it off and cast it from thee." In two patients, LSD had been used repeatedly, but one patient had used LSD only once.

References

1. Gerber JAD: Forensic pathology of drug related child abuse. In Wecht CH (ed): Legal Medical Annual, pp133–147. New York, Appleton-Century-Crofts, 1978
2. Mintz J, O'Brian CP, Pomerantz B: The threat of Viet Nam service on heroin addicted veterans. Am J Drug Alcohol Abuse 6:39–52, 1979
3. O'Brian CP, Nace EP, Mintz J, et al: The follow-up of Viet Nam veterans, relapse to drug use after Viet Nam service. Drug Alcohol Dependence 5:333–340, 1980
4. Robinson MG, Howe RC, Varni JG: Acute heroin withdrawal in Viet Nam. Clin Pharmacol Ther 16:303, 1974
5. Swertlow F: Hollywood's cocaine connection. TV Guide, February 28, 1981
6. Washtan AM, Stone NS: The human cost of chronic cocaine use. Medical Aspects of Human Sexuality 18:122–30, 1984
7. NY Times News Service, San Diego Union. September 16, 1979. Nichols JH: How opiates change behavior. Sci Am 212:80, 1965
8. Helpern M: Fatalities from narcotic addiction in New York City. Hum Pathol 3:13, 1972
9. Gage N: Cheap middle eastern heroin floods Europe, seeps into U.S. New York Times News Service, San Diego Union, January 3, 1980
10. Isbell H, et al: Chronic barbiturate intoxication. Arc Neurol Psychiatr 64:1, 1950
11. Montalbano WD: Latins push belated war on cocaine. Los Angeles Times, December 1, 1985, p 1
12. Alles GA: The comparative physiological action of phenylethanolamine. J Pharmacol Exp Ther 32:121, 1928
13. Welti CV, et al: Death caused by recreational cocaine use. JAMA 241:2519–2522, 1979
14. White L, et al: Intravenous propylhexedrine and sudden death. N Engl J Med 297:1071, 1977

15. Anderson RJ, et al: Intravenous propylhexedrine abuse and sudden death. Am J Med 67:15–20, 1979
16. Kessler JT, et al: Cerebral vasculitis in a drug abuser. J Clin Psychiatry 39:559–564, 1978
17. Meador KH, et al: Renal amyloidosis and subcutaneous drug abuse. An Int Med 91:565–567, 1979
18. Jacob H, et al: Amyloidosis secondary to drug abuse and chronic skin suppuration. Arch Int Med 138:1150–1151, 1978
19. Tindell TD: Intra-arterial injections of oral medications. N Engl J Med 287:1132–1133, 1972
20. Vega JM, et al: Rapidly spreading subcutaneous inflammation after "skin popping" in drug addicts. Am Surg 45:392–393, 1979
21. Aust NZ, Boughton CR, Hawkes RA: Viral hepatitis and the drug cult: A brief socioepidermological study in Sydney. Aust NZ J Med 10:157–161, 1980
22. Prevention of posttransfusion hepatitis. In Vyas, Dienstag, Hoofnagle (eds): Viral Hepatitis and Liver Disease, New York, Grune and Stratton, 1984
23. Dienstag JL, et al: Etiology of sporadic hepatitis B antigen-negative hepatitis. Ann Intern Med 87:1–6, 1977
24. Redeker AG: Delta agent and hepatitis B. Ann Int Med 98:542–543, 1983
25. Rarmondo, JR et al: Multicentre study of prevalence of HBV associated delta infection and liver disease in drug addicts. Lancet, 1982
26. Rezetto M: Hepatitis delta virus infection
27. Souri EN, Green WR: Intravitreal amphotericin B toxicity. Am J Ophthalmol 78:77–81, 1974
28. Center for Disease Control: Delta hepatitis—Mass. MMWR 33:493, 1984
29. Hilleman MR, et al: Hepatitis B and hepatitis A vaccines. In Szmuness W, et al (eds): Proceedings of an International Symposium on Viral Hepatitis, pp 385–397. 1981. Franklin Institute Press, 1982
30. Lange M, et al: Infective endocarditis in heroin addicts: Epidemiologic observations and some unusual cases. Am Heart J 96:144–152, 1978
31. Dishotsky NI, Loughman WD, Mogar RE, et al: LSD and genetic damage. Science 172:431–439, 1971
32. Benchimol A, et al: Accelerated ventricular rhythm and cocaine abuse. Ann Int Med 88:519–521, 1978
33. Ogbuawa O, et al: Comparison of staphylococcal and nonstaphylococcal endocarditis in narcotic addicts. South Med J 72:1557–1558, 1979
34. Crawford FA, et al: Tricuspid endocarditis in a drug addict. Chest 73:471–475, 1978
35. Marcus HR, et al: Eikenella corrodens subacute bacterial endocarditis. Mixed infection in amphetamine user. NYS J Med, December 1977, p 2261
36. Brandstetter RD, et al: Candida parapsilosis endocarditis. Recovery of the causative organism from an addict's own syringe. JAMA 243:1073, 1980
37. Harris PD, et al: Susceptibility of addicts to infection and neoplasia. N Engl J Med 286:310, 1972
38. Center for Disease Control: AIDS weekly surveillances report. MMWR 33:4–5, 1984
39. Center for Disease Control: Update on acquired immune deficiency syndrome (AIDS)—United States. MMWR 182:31:507–508, 513–514

40. Center for Disease Control Update: AIDS—U.S. MMWR 32:688–691, 1984
41. Masui H, et al: The acquired immune deficiency syndrome. In Remington and Swartz (eds): Current Clinical Topics in Infectious Diseases, New York, McGraw-Hill, 1985
42. Fugikawa LS, Salahuddin SZ, Palestine AG, et al: Isolation of human T-cell leukemia/lymphotrophic virus type III from the tears of a patient with acquired immune deficiency syndrome (AIDS). Lancet (in press)
43. Prot P, et al: AIDS in a heterosexual population in Zaire. Lancet 11:65–69, 1984
44. Michelson JB, et al: Foreign body granuloma of the retina associated with intravenous cocaine addiction. Am J Ophthalmol 87:278, 1979
45. Michelson JB, Freedman SB, Boyden DG: Aspergillus endophthalmitis in a drug abuser. Ann Ophthalmol 14:1051–1053, 1982
46. Francis CDC: Personal communication cited in Hollinger BF: Prevention of post transfusion hepatitis. In Viral Hepatitis and Liver Disease. Orlando, Grune & Stratton, 1984
47. Michelson JB: Color Atlas of Uveitis Diagnosis. Chicago, Yearbook Medical Publishers, 1984
48. McLane N, Carroll D: Ocular manifestations of drug abuse. Surv Ophthalmol 30:1–14, 1986
49. Mathiesen LR, et al: Epidemiology and clinical characteristics of acute hepatitis types A, B, and non-A, non-B. Scand J Gastroenterol 14:849–856, 1979
50. Jaffe J: Drug addiction and drug abuse. In Goodman LS, Gilman A: Pharmacologic Basis of Therapeutics, 5th ed. New York, Macmillan, 1975
51. Eddy NB, Halback H, Isbell H: Drug dependence: Its significance and characteristics. Bull WHO 32:721, 1965
52. Dole V: Narcotic addiction, physical dependence and relapse. N Engl J Med 286:988, 1972
53. Mintz J, O'Brian CP, Pomerantz B: The threat of Vietnam Service on heroin-addicted veterans. Am J Drug Alcohol Abuse 6:39–52, 1979
54. Center for Disease Control Update: AIDS—Europe. MMWR 33:607–609, 1984
55. Center for Disease Control: Unexplained immunodeficiency and opportunistic infections in infants. New York, New Jersey, California. MMWR 49:665–667, 1982
56. Rubenstein A, et al: Acquired immunodeficiency with reversed T_4/T_8 ratios in infants born to promiscuous and drug-addicted mothers. JAMA 249:2350, 1983
57. Brust JCM, Richter RW: Quinine amblyopia related to heroin addiction. Ann Int Med 74:84–86, 1971
58. Bard LA, Gills JP: Quinine amblyopia. Arch Ophthalmol 72:328–331, 1964
59. Burns RP, Steele A: Ocular changes in drug abusers. In Irving Legrold (ed): Symposium on Ocular Therapy, Vol 6. St. Louis, CV Mosby, 1973
60. Knox DL, Palmer CAL, English F: Iris atrophy after quinine amblyopia. Arch Ophthalmol 76:359–362, 1966
61. Lincoff MH: Quinine amblyopia. Arch Ophthalmol 53:382–385, 1955
62. Brown E, Meyer GG: Toxic amblyopia and peripheral neuropathy with ethchlorvyrol abuse. Am J Psychiatr 126:882–884, 1969
63. Haining WM, Beveridge GW: Toxic amblyopia in a patient receiving ethchlorvynol as a hypnotic. Br J Ophthalmol 48:598–600, 1964

64. Channer KS, Stanley S: Persistent visual hallucination secondary to chronic solvent encephelopathy. Neuro Neurosurg Psychiatr 46:83, 1983
65. Keane JR: Toluene optic neuropathy. Ann Neurol 4:390, 1978
66. Louria DB, Hensle T, Rose J: The major medical complications of heroin addiction. Ann Int Med 67:1–22, 1967
67. Aguilar GL, Blumenkranz MS, Egbert PR, et al: Candida endophthalmitis after intravenous drug abuse. Arch Ophthalmol 97:96–100, 1979
68. Elliott JH, O'Day DM, Cutow GS, et al: Mycotic endophthalmitis in drug abusers. Am J Ophthalmol 88:66–72, 1979
69. Getrick RA, Rodrigues MM: Endogenous fungal endophthalmitis in a drug addict. Am J Ophthalmol 77:680–683, 1974
70. Horne MJ, Ma MH, Taylor RF, et al: Candida endophthalmitis. Med J Aust 1:170–172, 1975
71. Salmon JF, Partridge BM, Spalton DJ: Candida endophthalmitis in a heroin addict: A case report. Br J Ophthalmol 67:306–309, 1983
72. Snip RC, Michels RG: Pars plana vitrectomy in the management of endogenous candida endophthalmitis. Am J Ophthalmol 5:699–704, 1976
73. Stern GA, Fetkenhour CL, O'Grady RB: Intravitreal amphotericin B treatment of Candida endophthalmitis. Arch Ophthalmol 95:89–93, 1977
74. Stone RD, Irvine AR, O'Connor GR: Candida endophthalmitis: Report of an unusual case with isolation of the etiologic agent by vitreous biopsy. Ann Ophthalmol 7:757–762, 1975
75. Sugar HS, Mandell GH, Shalev J: Metastatic endophthalmitis associated with injection of addictive drugs. Am J Ophthalmol 71:1055–1058, May 1971
76. Tarr KH: Candida endophthalmitis and drug abuse. Aust J Ophthalmol 8:303–305, 1980
77. Edwards JE Jr, Foos RY, Montgomrie JZ, et al: Ocular manifestations of candida septicemia: Review of 76 cases of hematogenous endophthalmitis. Medicine 53:47–75, 1974
78. Michelson JB, Freedman SD, Boyden DG: Aspergillus endophthalmitis in a drug abuser. Ann Ophthalmol 14:1051–1054, November 1982
79. Doft BH, Clarkson JC, Rebell G, et al: Endogenous aspergillus endophthalmitis in drug abusers. Arch Ophthalmol 98:859–862, 1980
80. Wilmarth SS, May DR, Roth AM, et al: Aspergillus endophthalmitis in an intravenous drug user. Ann Ophthalmol 15:470–476, 1983
81. Stenson S, Brookner A, Rosenthan S: Bilateral endogenous necrotizing scleritis due to Aspergillus oryzae. Ann Ophthalmol 14:62–72, January 1982
82. Dreyer NP, Fields BN: Heroin associated infective endocarditis. Ann Int Med 78:699–702, 1973
83. Lederer CM Jr, Sabates FN: Ocular findings in the intravenous drug abuser. Ann Ophthalmol 14:436–438, 1982
84. Banks T, Fletcher R, Ali N: Infective endocarditis in heroin addicts. Am J Med 55:444–451, 1973
85. Jarrett WH, Christy JH: Retinal hole formation from septic embolization in acute bacterial endocarditis. Am J Ophthalmol 64:472–474, 1967
86. Burns CL: Bilateral endophthalmitis in acute bacterial endocarditis. Am J Ophthalmol 88:909–913, 1979

87. Hatem G, Merritt JC, Cowan CC Jr: Bacillus cereus panophthalmitis following IV heroin. Ann Ophthalmol 11:431–440, March 1979
88. Masi RJ: Endogenous endophthalmitis associated with Bacillus cereus bacteremia in a cocaine addict. Ann Ophthalmol 10:1367–1370, October 1978
89. Young EY, Wallace RJ Jr, Ericsson CD, et al: Panophthalmitis due to Bacillus cereus. Arch Int Med 40:559–560, 1980
90. Limage SR, Goldberg MH: Septic submacular choroidal embolus associated with intravenous drug abuse. Ann Ophthalmol 14:518–522, June 1982
91. Eichner HL, Aebi E: Septic retinitis due to injection of a homemade alcoholic beverage. JAMA 213:1644–1646, 1970
92. Fauci AS, Macher AM, Longo DL, et al: Acquired immunodeficiency syndrome: Epidemiologic, clinical, immunologic and therapeutic considerations. Ann Int Med 100:92–106, 1984
93. Gottlieb MS, Groopman JE, Weinstein WM, et al: The acquired immunodeficiency syndrome. Ann Int Med 99:208–220, 1983
94. Gottlieb MS, Schroft R, Schanker HM, et al: Pneumocystis carini pneumonia and mucosal candidiasis in previously healthy homosexual men: Evidence of a new acquired cellular immunodeficiency. N Engl J Med 305:1425–1431, 1981
95. Holland GN, Pepose JS, Pettit TH, et al: Acquired immune deficiency syndrome, ocular manifestations. Ophthalmology 90:859–873, 1983
96. Newman NM, Mendel MR, Gullett J, et al: Clinical and histologic findings in opportunistic ocular infections: Part of a new syndrome of acquired immunodeficiency. Arch Ophthalmol 101:396–401, 1983
97. Palestine AG, Rodrigues MM, Macher AM, et al: Ophthalmic involvement in acquired immunodeficiency syndrome. Ophthalmology 91:1092–1099, 1984
98. Pepose JS, Nestor MS, Holland GN: An analysis of retinal cotton-wool spots and cytomegalovirus retinitis in acquired immunodeficiency syndrome. Am J Ophthalmol 95:118–120, 1983
99. Rosenberg PR, Uliss AE, Friedland GH, et al: Acquired immunodeficiency syndrome: Ophthalmic manifestations in ambulatory patients. Ophthalmology 90:874–878, 1983
100. Sadun AC, Sadun AA, Sadun LA: Solar retinopathy: A biophysical analysis. Arch Ophthalmol 102:1510–1512, 1984
101. Council on Scientific Affairs: The acquired immunodeficiency syndrome. JAMA 252:2037–2043, 1984
102. Brucker AJ: Disc and peripheral retinal neovascularization secondary to talc and cornstarch emboli. Am J Ophthalmol 88:864–867, 1979
103. Friburg TR, Gragoudas ES, Rejan COT: Talc emboli and macular ischemia in intravenous drug abuse. Arch Ophthalmol 97:1089–1091, 1979
104. Schatz H, Drake M: Self-injected retinal emboli. Ophthalmology 86:468–485, 1979
105. Siepser SB, Magargal LE, Augsburger JJ: Acute bilateral retinal microembolism in a heroin addict. Ann Ophthalmol 13:699–702, 1981
106. Murphy SB, Jackson WB, Pare JAP: Talc retinopathy. Can J Ophthalmol 13:152, 1978
107. Keane JR: Embolic retinopathy from carotid artery self-injection. J Clin Neuro-ophthalmol 1:119–121, 1981

108. Lee J, Spira JD: Retinal and cerebral microembolization of talc in a drug abuser. Am J Med 265:75–77, 1973
109. Kresca LJ, Goldberg MF, Jampol LM: Talc emboli and retinal neovascularization in a drug abuser. Am J Ophthalmol 87:334–339, 1979
110. Tse DT, Ober RR: Talc retinopathy. Am J Ophthalmol 90:624–640, 1980
111. Jampol LM, Setogawa T, Rednam KRV, et al: Talc retinopathy in primates. A model of ischemic retinopathy: I. Clinical Studies. Arch Ophthalmol 99:1273–1280, 1981
112. Bluth LL, Hanscom TA: Retinal detachment and vitreous hemorrhage due to talc emboli. JAMA 246:980–981, 1981
113. Fuller DG: Severe solar maculopathy associated with the use of lysergic acid diethylamide (LSD). Am J Ophthalmol 81:413–416, 1976
114. Binegar GN, Wolter JR: Marijuana smoking, sun gazing, central scotomas and steroids. J Ped Ophthalmol Strubismus 8:98–101, 1971
115. Ewald RA: Sun gazing associated with the use of LSD. Ann Ophthalmol 3:15–17, 1971
116. Rosen DH, Hoffman AM: Focal suicide: Self enucleation by two young psychotic individuals. Am J Psychiatr 128:1009–1012, 1972
117. Thomas RB, Fuller DH: Self-inflicted ocular injury associated with drug abuse. J SC Med Assoc 68:202–203, 1972

TEN

Inflammatory Retinal Detachment

Uveitis in retinal detachment can be related in three ways: (1) exudative retinal detachment can be a component of the underlying uveitis (Fig. 10-1); (2) uveitis can be a late complication of chronic rhegmatogenous retinal detachment; (3) rhegmatogenous or retinal detachment due to traction can be a complication of uveitis (Figs. 10-2, 10-3).

Differential Diagnosis

It is of paramount importance to determine whether a uveitic retinal detachment is caused by subretinal serous exudation, traction due to contracting postinflammatory vitreous bands, or a break (hole) in the retina. In certain diseases such as Vogt-Koyanagi-Harada syndrome or posterior scleritis, secondary exudative retinal detachments may frequently occur (see Fig. 10-1). Affected patients are *not* surgical candidates, unless the detachment is of such a long-standing and refractory nature that retinal necrosis from ischemia is feared, in which case drainage must be considered. A situation may arise where diagnosis is achieved only by ultrasonography (see Figs. 10-2, 10-3); for example the opacity of uveitic cataract or of very dense vitritis may preclude ophthalmoscopic visualization. Such a case is noted in Fig. 10-2, a patient with Behçet's disease with profoundly dense vitritis and traction retinal detachment noted by ultrasound alone. Symptoms were

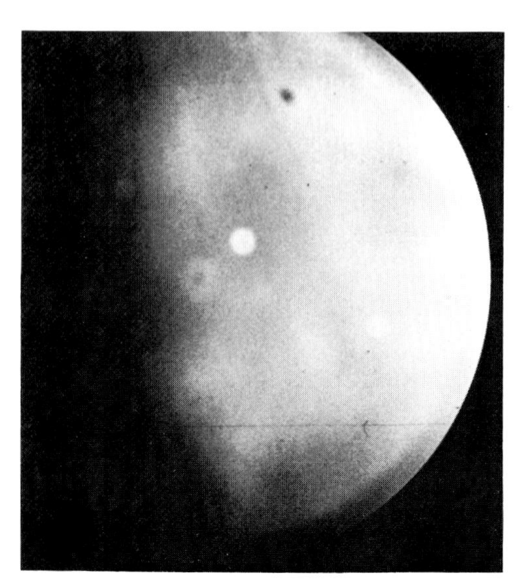

Figure 10-1. Ophthalmoscopic appearance of exudative retinal detachment in a patient with Vogt-Koyanagi-Harada disease. Note the extensive fluid under the retina and the accompanying vasculitis in the retina itself.

suggested by the patient himself who noted dramatic and abrupt vision loss, but ophthalmoscopy was precluded because of the dense intra-ocular inflammation even though retinal detachment was suspected. It was this "sticky" inflammation alone that caused retinal traction and consequent detachment. Pars plana vitrectomy may be necessary first, merely to examine the retina and second, to achieve a release of retinal traction. Such a situation is seen with those uveitides, such as Behçet's disease, Vogt-Koyanagi-Harada disease, toxoplasmosis, endophthalmitis, or sympathetic ophthalmia (Fig. 10-4), which produce profound vitreous inflammation or hemorrhage. Rarely does anterior segment inflammation cause such a problem. Table 10-1 lists conditions in which there may be a combination of intra-ocular inflammation (uveitis) and retinal detachment.

Serous or exudative retinal detachments characteristically present with shifting fluid, absence of holes, and absence of significant traction. Vogt-Koyanagi-Harada syndrome is a classic inflammatory disease characterized by serous retinal detachment (see Fig. 10-1). Rarely is sympathetic ophthalmia accompanied by similar exudation. A localized serous elevation, as opposed to the multiloculated elevation of the Vogt-Koyanagi-Harada syndrome, may accompany the severe posterior scleritis and uveitis associated with rheumatoid arthritis. Any severe retinitis (e.g., tuberculous or syphilitic) can cause secondary retinal holes, severe toxoplasmic retinochoroiditis, pars planitis, and even Behçet's disease with vasculitis may sometimes be associated with exudation, traction, or rhegmatogenous detachment (Figs. 10-4, 10-5, 10-6) and pars planitis may be associated

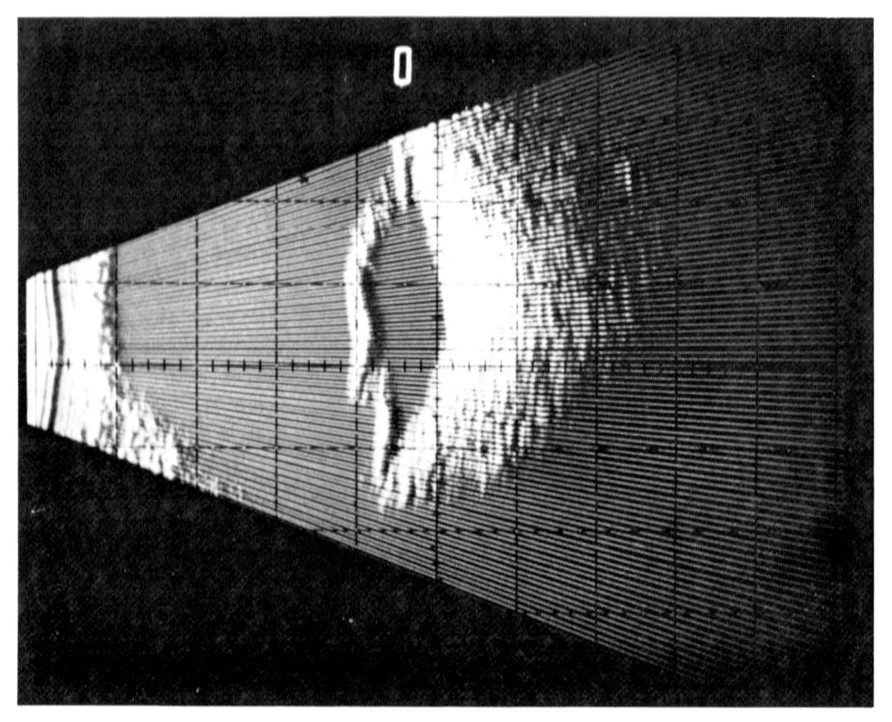

Figure 10-2. B-scan ultrasonogram demonstrating large bullous retinal detachment caused by "sticky" reaction from thickened, inflamed vitreous, which precludes ophthalmoscopy in this patient with Behçet's disease.

with progressive traction or rhegmatogenous detachment over a long period of time. An extreme and acute example is the acute retinal necrosis syndrome, which eventuates in both phenomena and consequently yields a dramatically poor result from surgery. In such cases, vitrectomy is necessary to eliminate the vitreous gel; its fibrous and "sticky" components lead to traction and tear formation. External scleral buckling is often needed as well to "close the holes" and reduce traction. Some purely traction detachments are resolved with vitrectomy alone by releasing the adhesive inflammatory bands that elevate the sensory retina. Excessive tissue manipulation should be avoided because such maneuvers may contribute to the late development of massive periretinal proliferation on an inflammatory basis, or in the short run may cause retinal pulling and pushing, and contribute to further tear and hole formation.

Clinical Features

Patients with uveitis and retinal detachment have all the clinical signs and symptoms of both disorders. If the retina is totally detached, central as well as periph-

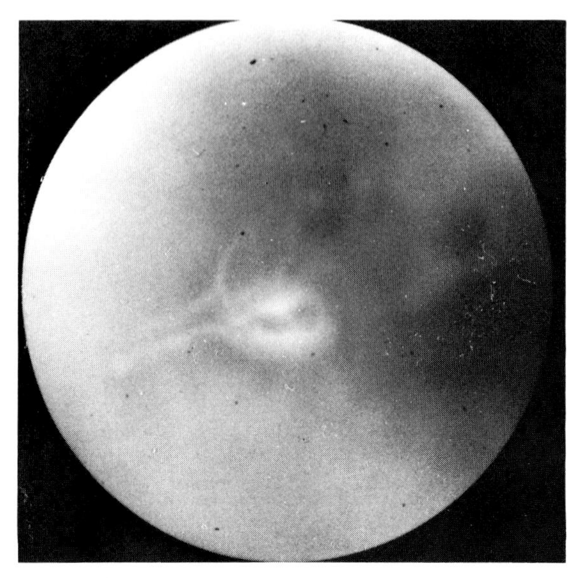

Figure 10-3. Fundus photograph of the patient in Figure 10-2, whose thickened and turbid vitreous, with chronic Behçet's disease, precluded visualization of "sticky" traction retinal detachment of the macula and supratemporal retina as seen in the ultrasonogram.

eral vision is lessened or lost; if it is only partially detached, the usual complaints are a shower of spots and floaters, a delineated blind spot or, in cases of secondary traction or rhegmatogenous detachment, a cloud-like or curtain-like veil obstructing the vision.

Nearly every patient with noninflammatory retinal detachment shows a *slight* degree of anterior uveitis evidenced by flare and cells in the aqueous. This must be differentiated from the frankly active uveitis patient whose ocular inflammation becomes complicated by the formation of retinal breaks and retinal detachment. Occasionally, a retinal detachment with acute uveitis is accompanied by fibrous exudates and either secondary glaucoma or, more usually, severe hypotony. The pressure may be at the level of only 1 or 2 mm Hg. When hypotony is present, massive choroidal detachments simulating a choroidal melanoma can be seen. In rare instances, an unsuspected intra-ocular foreign body may be responsible for both the uveitis and the retinal detachment (see Chapter 11). For example, an exudative retinal detachment may be seen combined with rhegmatogenous detachment, both resulting from undetected steel foreign body in the choroid or retina (see Chapter 11). Ultrasonography of the orbit and gonioscopy should be performed on all patients with active uveitis associated with any retinal detachment to rule out the possibility of an unsuspected intraocular foreign body.

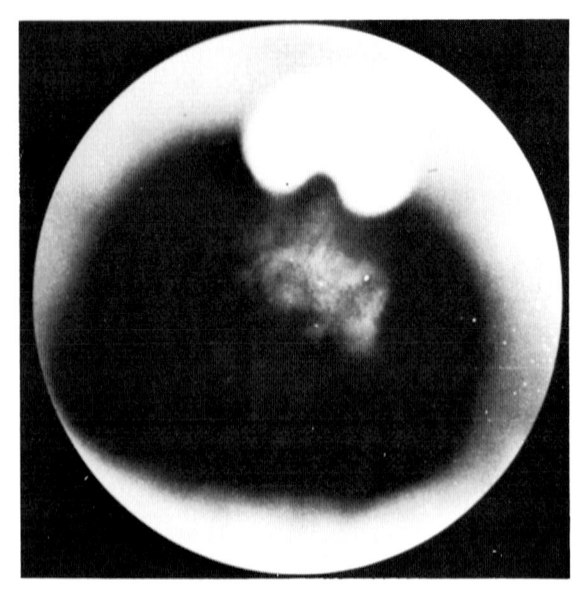

Figure 10-4. Fundus photograph showing original focus of retinitis of atrophic retina where zoster retinitis caused rhegmatogenous detachment, is now sitting on scleral buckle all the intended signs of inflammation.

Patients with retinal detachment who are not receiving strong midriatics prior to surgery may develop posterior synechiae as a result of the mild uveitis that nearly always accompanies even retinal detachment without a uveitis syndrome. These synechiae interfere with ophthalmoscopy and localization of retinal breaks. It is often important to use a midriatic such as neo-synephrine, which can "bounce" the pupil rather than dilating the pupil widely. Even without uveitis and owing to the low level of intra-ocular inflammation that is often present with uncomplicated retinal detachment alone, atropine may serve to form synechiae and fasten the pupil down in the dilated position. This, of course, will lead to a profound photophobia for the retinal detachment patient in the postoperative period.

When uveitis causes marked flare and cells with keratic precipitates and multiple synechiae, it may be necessary to postpone retinal surgery. An operation performed during active inflammation may be complicated by intra-ocular hemorrhage and marked stimulation of the uveitis. After basic laboratory investigation is undertaken to detect a possible etiologic factor, treatment of uveitis should include specific therapy for cases of known origin. For example, patients with retinal detachment secondary to toxoplasmosis that has been in the active phase (toxoplasmosis "eats" a hole in the retina from the reactivated lesions causing rhegmatogenous detachment (Fig. 10-7), should be treated with the full

TABLE 10-1. Retinal Detachments and the Types of Uveitis With Which They May Be Associated

Type of Detachment	Type of Uveitis
Serous (exudative)	Vogt-Koyanagi-Harada syndrome
	Sympathetic ophthalmia
	Posterior scleritis (rheumatoid arthritis)
	Toxoplasmic retinochoroiditis
Traction	Toxoplasmic retinochoroiditis
	Pars planitis
	Behçet's disease
	Any severe retinitis
Rhegmatogenous	Toxoplasmic retinochoroiditis
	Pars planitis
	Behçet's disease
	Any severe retinitis (e.g., acute retinal necrosis syndrome, CMV retinitis)

regimen for toxoplasmosis as well as with "heavy duty" immunosuppressives. This approach is necessary in order to lessen the inflammatory impediment to (1) the surgical stage of the procedure, which of course can lead to massive periretinal proliferation, and (2) the postsurgical period where healing in the absence of

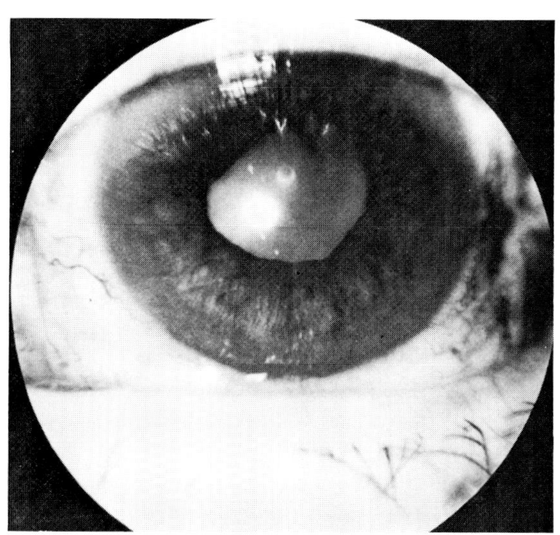

Figure 10-5. External view of an eye demonstrating dense vitreal inflammation secondary to reactivated toxoplasmosis in which a traction retinal detachment occurred. Fundus photography was precluded by the thick exudate.

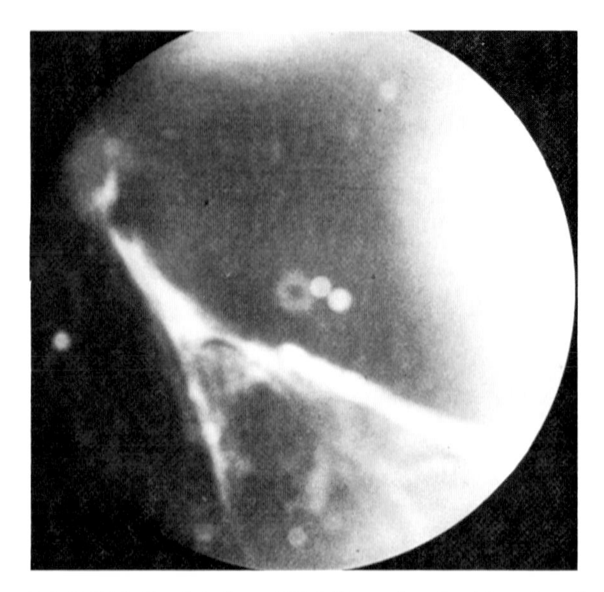

Figure 10-6. Fundus view of thick fibrous bands with profound intravitreal inflammation due to reactivated toxoplasmosis with combined traction/rhegmatogenous retinal detachment.

inflammation is so important (Fig. 10-8). In addition, midriatics four or more times a day, and 1% prednisolone sodium phosphate drops every 1 to 2 hours should be used. High doses of oral prednisone (100 mg) may be prescribed daily until after the retinal operation. The dose is then gradually reduced to 30 mg or 40 mg per day until the inflammation caused by the retina surgery as well as the presurgical underlying disorder subsides. It is also cogent to consider the use of periocular steroids in this surgical phase.

Active chorioretinitis or retinitis of long duration can cause considerable vitreous haze. When affected with retinal detachment in addition, such an eye may create problems in management. If vitreous opacities due to either inflammation or hemorrhage prevent adequate diagnosis and treatment of the retinal detachment, the uveitis must be treated first. A closed vitrectomy may be needed as a primary operation to clear the vitreous, followed by scleral buckling operation later when deemed appropriate.

Pars Planitis—"Intermediate Cyclitis"

Pars planitis, intermediate cyclitis, or peripheral uveitis is a clinical entity first described by Schepens in 1950.[1,2] It deserves special mention as a dual phenomenon with continuous low-grade inflammation and possible progressive long-term retinal traction, and then detachment. It affects both sexes equally and is bilateral in approximately 75% of the cases. The disease usually starts at an early age and is

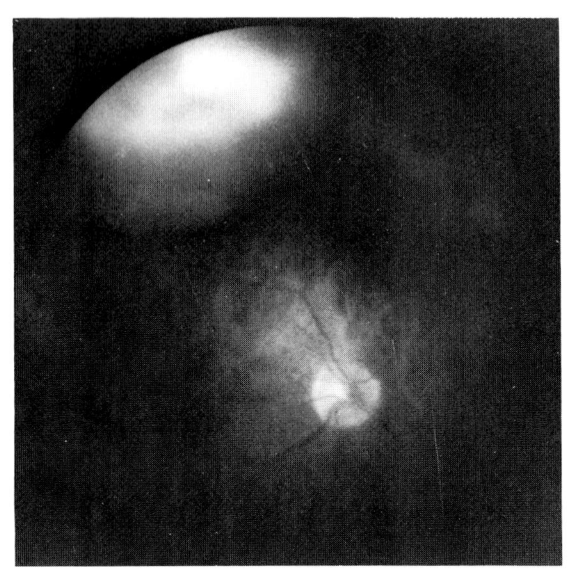

Figure 10-7. After vitrectomy and scleral buckling note the etiologic epiretinal lesion at the 11:30 position on the buckle, now inactive. (The patient's serum IFA toxoplasmosis titer was 1:1024 at surgery; the vitrectomy fluid yielded a titer of 1:4096.)

progressive. It may be noted in infancy, more frequently in adolescence, and usually begins at age 20 to 30 years. We know that the disease tends to "burn itself out" after 10 or 15 years of active inflammation. If the patients are left with none of the serious sequelae of the disease at the time of "burn-out" (i.e., cataract, glaucoma, or, most important, a sclerotic-type cystoid macular edema), they may possess good vision and have little complication from it. The inception of the intra-ocular inflammation is either silent or accompanied by minimal symptoms of blurred vision, "tiredness in the eyes," or floaters. By the time the condition is diagnosed, however, serious visual loss may be present in almost one half of the cases.[3]

Fundus changes in the early stages may be limited to preretinal aggregates of exudative material in the vicinity of the ora serrata. These yellowish-gray globular exudates may be found on the inner surface of the pars plana ciliaris at the ora serrata or on the anterior portion of the retina. Often, but not always, they are located on the course of peripheral retinal vessels and the signs of perivasculitis (most often periphlebitis) are evidenced at the terminal retinal vessels by sheathing and obliteration. This clinical picture may simulate the presentation of sarcoidosis in the peripheral retinal. As this inflammatory process continues, the exudative deposits may coalesce to form a massive snow bank that covers the ora serrata region, hiding normal landmarks there. In the ongoing stages of inflammation, these deposits may vascularize and may rupture and hemorrhage. This

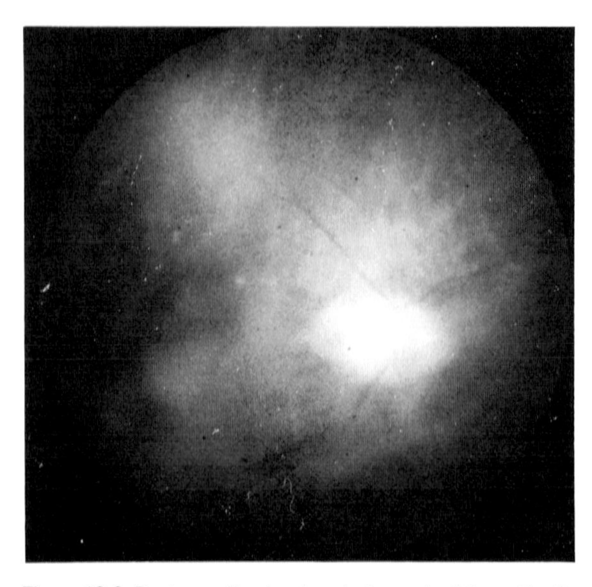

Figure 10-8. Postoperative fundus photograph of the patient in Figure 10-2 during "boggy" edematous retina, now "snapped" back into its restored, flat position, after the burden of "sticky" tractional elements of the vitreous inflammatory bands have been lysed and removed.

vascularization may cause not only vitreous hemorrhage in the pars plana or beyond but also tears and holes in the retina leading to rhegmatogenous as well as traction detachment from these "sticky masses" in the peripheral retina (Fig. 10-9).

Exudative material may appear in the vitreous cavity where it forms white or yellowish "cotton balls" located close to the retina. It is at this stage that the macula often develops its cystoid edema. In time, degeneration in the retinal pigment epithelium may develop as well. Twenty percent of cases may show gel-like exudation on the trabeculum, and a mild trabeculitis may ensue with secondary glaucoma. Exudation on the anterior iris surface may produce adhesions between the iris and trabeculum.[4]

The course of the disease is variable. In severe cases, which are rare, the perivasculitis may be a prominent feature, and all the retinal blood vessels including the arteries may gradually close. In some few extreme cases the process is acute, and both eyes may become blind with vasculitis and optic atrophy within months. The more frequent course of events in severe cases is the development of a cyclitic membrane, as is seen in juvenile rheumatoid arthritis. This is particularly frequent in the more juvenile form of the disease; whereas vascular occlusion is usually seen in the adult, progressing from the peripheral retina toward the disc, eventually obliterating most of the vasculature, simulating a clinical presentation

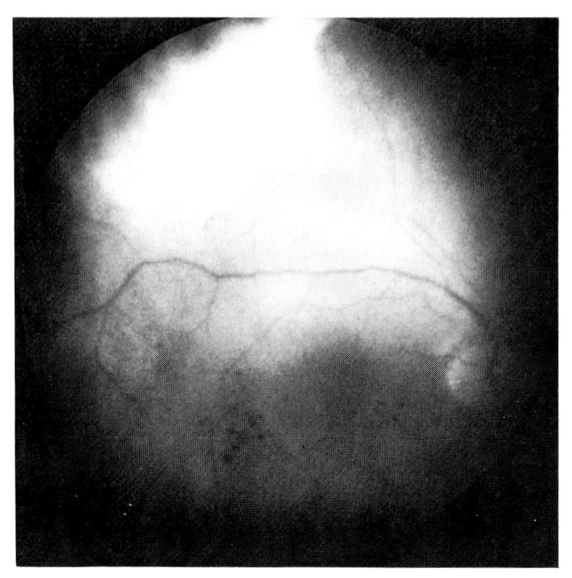

Figure 10-9. Patient with herpes zoster ophthalmicus and herpetic retinitis demonstrating an atrophic area in the retina of inflammation, which later "will have eaten through" the retina, causing a rhegmatogenous detachment.

of retinal necrosis as seen in sarcoid, connective tissue disease, or acute retinal necrosis (ARN).

Several types of retinal detachment occur prominently in pars planitis either alone or in combination. Exudative retinal detachment with choroidal detachment may be a prominent feature. Retinal detachment caused by traction without retinal breaks may be seen, or a frankly rhegmatogenous retinal detachment, due to one or several retinal tears in the very peripheral retina adjacent to snow banking, may be seen more frequently.

The very benign form of pars planitis usually progresses slowly, with many remissions and exacerbations, and becomes quiescent at an early stage. However, the data put forth by Schepens show that 40% of cases of pars planitis exhibit some degree of rhegmatogenous retinal detachment, sometimes bilaterally. During the early phase of active peripheral disease, symptoms are minimal and occasionally absent. Inactive inflammatory exudates are observed overlying the peripheral fundus along the ora serrata. Patients may complain solely of minimal "floaters." The retina often may show a zone of white "with or without pressure" that represents an increase in optical density of the retina as a consequence of thickening and edema, as well as a slight elevation of the retina due to traction by the vitreous body, which is undergoing syneresis in some portions and consolidation in others as a result of the increase in vitreous opacities. In the later phases, active exudation over the pars plana, especially inferiorly, is replaced by a thick white membrane that is often so dense that the ora serrata cannot be observed through it. This white membrane may coalesce and "heap up" into the prominent "snow bank" of pars planitis. This snow bank may be responsible for progressive retinal detachment. Pigmented demarcation lines form because the detachment remains stationary during long periods of time in the slowly progressive form of the disease. In some cases it is equally likely that invisible retinal breaks exist, hidden under the white membrane and the white snow bank.

Many of the patients in this group are children who, characteristically, often fail to notice and report the gradual loss of upper visual field caused by the progression of the retinal detachment and may not seek medical advice until essential vision has been lost for weeks or months. For this reason and because retinal detachment may be such a prominent form of even the benign part of pars planitis, it is important to examine the fundus of known uveitis patients, especially children, at least twice a year. This examination should include careful scrutiny of the entire fundus periphery with scleral depression. Generally, eyes affected in this fashion respond well to surgery for retinal detachment. There is very little intercurrent inflammation, such as that seen in the other uveitides like toxoplasmosis, acute retinal necrosis, cytomegalovirus infection, which would be a poor prognostic index for the surgical procedure. These patients do extremely well with an encircling element (scleral buckle) without the need for vitrectomy; although if prominent traction is noted, certainly the treatment of choice is vitrectomy, and vitrectomy alone, where traction alone is responsible for the detachment phenomenon (Fig. 10-10).

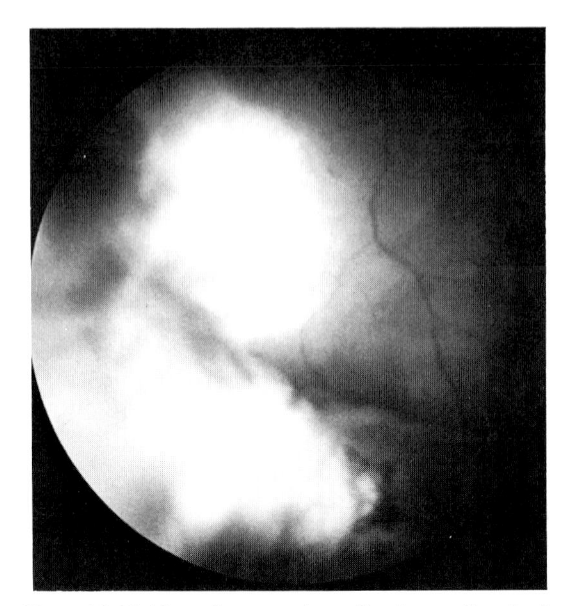

Figure 10-10. View after pars plana vitrectomy with scleral buckling shows a scleral buckle below and one dumbbell-shaped prior lesion of active toxoplasmosis at the 8:00 position.

A more severe but still mild type of peripheral uveitis smolders for years with exacerbations and remissions. In what Schepens would describe as "mild peripheral uveitis," 50% of cases develop rhematogenous retinal detachment due to tears and holes in the retinal periphery, usually contiguous with and adjacent to the snow banking and white membranes in the peripheral retina, especially inferiorly.[12] As a consequence of the chronicity and low activity of uveitis, membrane formation tends to be marked in the area of the vitreous base, especially where exudation is most abundant. Vitreous shrinkage may be pronounced, resulting in larger retinal breaks than those that occur in the more benign type of pars planitis. Fixed retinal folds may also be frequent. The proliferation that leads to the membrane formation and organization of the vitreous base may extend posteriorly over the retinal breaks, effectively sealing them and preventing the further development of retinal detachment, while in other instances macular edema develops and subretinal fluid accumulates gradually under retinal breaks before the membrane can seal it. The detached retina may appear cystic, resembling a retinoschisis, and large breaks may be produced, resembling dialyses at the vitreous base contiguous to the membrane formation at the ora. When a true retinal dialysis is observed, without signs of pars planitis, in a young patient in the absence of trauma, it may be difficult to determine whether or not this is the result of mild chronic pars planitis. Helpful diagnostic signs are the retinal periphlebitis and vasculitis in the periphery; fresh exudates in the fundus periphery, vitreous, or filtration angle, and the signs of pars planitis in the fellow eye.

Surgery for retinal detachment is often well tolerated in this type of case, and scleral buckling without vitrectomy may do very well. The damage to the vitreous base by the inflammatory process may cause insidious vitreous shrinkage. If this is the case, a scleral buckling alone is indicated. Patients with these milder types of chronic pars planitis should be followed usually at 4 to 6 month intervals. If breaks without retinal detachment are observed when the uveitis remains only slightly active, it is best to treat the retinal breaks with laser or cryopexy. One may even postpone and carefully watch the development of such breaks, since the proliferating membrane at the vitreous base and over the ora may seal the breaks by itself in time. When a clinical rhegmatogenous detachment occurs and extends posteriorly to the equator, with resultant visual field defect, surgery is necessary.

Severe Pars Planitis

Cases of very severe pars planitis are characterized by neovascularization arising anterior to the ora serrata, apparently from the ciliary body, and growing posteriorly into the exudates. With the passage of months or years, the fundus periphery simultaneously shows areas of active inflammation and organization of the vitreous base. The neovascularization that occurs may rupture and hemorrhage causing vitreous hemorrhage, thus causing further vitreous shrinkage and contraction and, of course, even more traction on the retina. This then becomes a vicious cycle: more hemorrhages, more vitreous shrinkage, more contraction forces on the vitreous base, more retinal traction. If neovascularization of the vitreous base at the snow banks is noted, the use of cryopexy for this as originally advocated by Aaberg[1] is a treatment of choice. It is of interest that his original advocacy was limited to the development of new snow banks only on the inferior portion of the peripheral retina and had nothing to do with the development of neovascularization.

Often this newly formed inflammatory tissue grows circumferentially converting the vitreous base to an annulus of scar tissue, much as is seen more posteriorly in diabetes. Large inferior retinal breaks develop posteriorly to the organized exudation. Horseshoe tears may now be found superiorly as well as inferiorly, and retinal detachment is said to develop in about 60% of such cases of severe progressive pars planitis. The detachment progresses rapidly and is usually accompanied by fixed retinal folds. Other examples of severe uveitis complicated by this type of progressive inexorable retinal detachment may include toxoplasmosis in the active stage with fibrous band formation, and its concurrent "hot" inflammation in the focus of reactivation may "eat" holes in the retina. *Toxocara canis* infection, with its fixed retinal folds from the periphery to the optic papilla, may do the same; and the active stage of endophthalmitis, with its developing fixed retinal folds prestaging the inexorable events for "massive periretinal proliferation" or "progressive vitreous retinopathy," may do this also. Acute retinal necrosis, the most severe and profound example of this phenomenon of progressive uveitis with rhegmatogenous and traction retinal detachment, poses the greatest risk to vision. All the components of treatment and surgery that have been mentioned so far are usually unsuccessful in these latter cases.

Surgery is usually poorly tolerated when intra-operative and postoperative inflammation is poorly controlled. Since the flare-up of the uveitis complicates a surgical intervention and often is the stimulus for massive periretinal proliferation, systemic steroids of maximum dose should be given for 2 days before operation (at least 60 mg to 120 mg of prednisone in adults, depending on body weight), during operation, and in the early postoperative period. If uveitis continues to be active, the therapy may be maintained and then withdrawn gradually until after the intra-ocular inflammation has been controlled. Other immunosuppressives may be added to the regimen.

Because severe chronic peripheral uveitis is accompanied by neovascularization and organization of the vitreous base, traction on the retina is marked and will continue in the future, even in the postoperative period, unless *all* of the vitreous has been removed and severed from its base. A core vitrectomy is insufficient, since circumferential traction can still remain. In such cases, permanent scleral buckling with the encircling silicon band is always used to relieve whatever additional traction there may be at the vitreous base. Some of these cases will be relentlessly progressive in spite of scleral buckling and full vitrectomy and may follow a rapid course, always ending in total retinal detachment, hypotony, and phthisis. The process is associated with a marked degree of peripheral neovascularization and macular edema. This has also been the outcome in almost all cases of acute retinal necrosis. Within a few months, severe organization of the exudate occurs and a cicatrizing annulus forms in the vitreous base. The damaged vitreous body shrinks, pulls the retina off, and marked thick folds, which often extend from the peripheral annulus to the optic nerve head, lead to "progressive vitreo-retinopathy." This forms so-called morning glory "cardboard" end-stage retinal detachment. Often no retinal breaks can even be found in this end stage, although surely they occur, because they are obscured by the exudates in the vitreous membranes. This end result of a totally fixed and inoperable retinal detachment often has telltale signs of a chronic periperal uveitis of lesser violence and useful vision in the fellow eye. However, one must remember also to watch for all of the signs and stigmata of sympathetic ophthalmia, which can ensue even up to 20 years after all of the profound damage has occurred to the most affected eye.

Other signs of relentlessly progressive end-stage uveitis with retinal detachment include lens opacity, which may occur soon after the operation, and phthisis bulbi with rapid shrinkage of the globe, which often leaves the patient with a cosmetically unacceptable appearance. The rapid progression of this disease phenomenon is not appreciably altered by the use of steroids administered locally or systemically.

Association of Rhegmatogenous and Exudative Retinal Detachment

About 6% to 8% of normal eyes have clinically silent retinal breaks. Occasionally an exudative retinal detachment or a uveal effusion may develop in such an eye. This is most common in Vogt-Koyanagi-Harada disease, sympathetic ophthalmia, and the uveal effusion syndrome, where clinically silent retinal breaks may have been present prior to the development of exudative retinal detachment. If the area of the retinal break is affected by the nonrhegmatogenous retinal detachment, a rhegmatogenous detachment becomes superimposed upon it, much as occurs with retinal detachment when it rarely becomes superimposed over retinoschisis. Generally it is not difficult to recognize such a superimposition. Indications of exudative disease are the signs of uveitis with flare, cells and, fibrinous outpouring in the anterior chamber; keratic precipitates; marked flare and cells in the fluid portion of the vitreous often "out-of-proportion" to a rhegmatogenous detachment. There also may be inflammatory precipitates on the detached hyaloid face, vasculitis of the retinal vessels, choroidal elevations and detachments, and hypotony. One must remember that any amount of vitreous hemorrhage may occur in association with noninflammatory rhegmatogenous retinal detachment alone and the pigmented nature of these cells may not be appreciated on lamp ophthalmoscopy. The cells may be confused with what might be supposed to be coexistent intra-ocular inflammation. The presence of signs of exudative uveitis without retinal breaks in the fellow eye may help to establish a diagnosis, especially where the "typical footprints" of recurrent exudative retinal detachment with scarring and pigment dispersion, hypo- and hyperpigmentary changes of inflammation of the retinal pigment epithelium are obvious. In the case of concomitant uveal effusion or of primary choroidal detachment, the signs of inflammation usually are minimal inside the eye and the correct diagnosis may be more difficult.

There are other situations in which a rhegmatogenous retinal detachment shows choroidal detachment pre-operatively and in which profound hypotony may occur. Some of these may have a similar pathogenesis to the uveal effusion syndrome. In some cases rhegmatogenous retinal detachment alone could induce a mild exudative or transudative retinal and choroidal detachment. In Vogt-Koyanagi-Harada disease the existence of the retinal tears may be pre-existent to the exudative detachment or may be due to tractional forces. The prognosis for surgery in such a case is poor.

When exudative and rhegmatogenous retinal detachments appear to be associated, the cause of the uveitis should be sought. The possibility of exacerbation by an undetected foreign body in the eye should not be neglected, and ultrasonography and gonioscopy should always be included in the workup of such a patient. Presence of a spontaneous choroidal detachment at the time of operation makes the surgical prognosis poor and the operation difficult, especially when pars plana vitrectomy is a concomitant of the surgery. Chorioretinal scarring and reaction must be monitored very carefully with minimal treatments, considering both cryoapplication and diathermy, for fear of provoking even further intra-ocular inflammation. Occasionally a choroidal tap may be entertained to reduce choroidal effusion and hemorrhage in such cases, especially where choroidal effusion may preclude the introduction of instruments for pars plana vitrectomy. While a choroidal effusion may be considered "Mother Nature's buckle" to help push the retinal pigment epithelium and the choroid up against the detached retina, it can often interfere dangerously with pre-operative procedures and postoperative healing. If choroidal effusion should resolve faster than the sequelae of the retinal detachment, one may be left with increasing fluid under the retina, after the choroidal has absorbed, suddenly leaving the tears and holes unbuckled and "open."

The sclera is usually thickened and edematous in these cases, and itself may be responsible for "leaking fluid" and holding sutures poorly. It is inadvisable to cut a scleral bed for a buckle in such cases since the undermining is often edematous and leaky, and the choroid itself is usually inflamed and may even be frankly hemorrhagic. An exoplant is preferred. One may consider the pre-operative use of photocoagulation around the tears and breaks rather than cryoapplication or diathermy to the outside of the eye, when this is applicable, since the thickened sclera may not allow for the penetration of the artificial "irritant" desirable for an adequate chorioretinal adhesion. These patients should continue to receive intensive steroid therapy until their excessive inflammation (caused by the retina operation as well as their intra-ocular inflammation) has been controlled (see Figs. 10-9 and 10-10).

Herpetic Retinitis

The increasing occurrence of acquired immune deficiency syndrome (AIDS) has caused an increase in the number of cases of herpetic retinitis. Whereas cytomegalic inclusion disease retinitis, and, less commonly, *Herpes zoster,* was once routinely associated with exogenous immunosuppression from organ transplantation or cancer therapy, its clinical setting has changed and its frequency has increased along with the explosive increase in drug abuse in the United States. With the epidemic of AIDS it is mandatory that any young person who presents with the typical hemorrhagic, exudative, necrosing retinitis of CMV should be considered to be a drug abuser, or to have AIDS, or both, until proven otherwise (see Chap. 9).

Although this intensely necrosing retinitis may present beyond the limits of medical/surgical treatment, both rhegmatogenous and/or traction retinal detachment from inflammation may occur. While the severity of necrosis in the retina may mitigate against a scleral buckle, the preferred mode of repair is vitrectomy with air gas (SF_6, C_3F_8) bubble tamponade.

The medical treatment of *Herpes simplex* retinitis, CMV retinitis, and *Varicella zoster* retinitis currently specifies acyclovir, 1500 mg/kg intravenously twice a day for 10 to 14 days, with 75 μm intravitreal. Gancyclovir (DHPG), 5 mg/kg intravenously twice a day for 14 to 21 days, with follow-up 60 mg/kg/day intravenously for 5 to 7 days (intra-ocular dose, 200 μm, once or twice a week) may also be given. Both acyclovir and gancyclovir are guanosine derivatives.

Miscellaneous

Cryopexy and photocoagulation have found limited application in the control of intra-ocular inflammation. While Aaberg[1] has advocated their use in the treatment of the pars plana in chronic cyclitis, the method is seldom used except for neovascularization of the snow banks. Similarly, cryopexy[2] and photocoagulation[8,9] have not gained widespread acceptance in the treatment of active toxoplasmic retinochoroiditis lesions. New immunologic treatments, such as plasmapheresis, have been reported to eliminate the burden of immune-complex deposition from the blood[10] in cases of known immune-mediated vasculitis (i.e., Behçet's disease). The increasing pursuit of new applications of intra-ocular microsurgery coupled with the ever expanding vista of immunologic mechanisms should make the future ever more promising for both the patient with uveitis and the ophthalmologist.

References

1. Aaberg TM, Cesarz TJ, Flikinger RR: Treatment of peripheral uveoretinitis by cryotherapy. Am J Ophthalmol 75:685, 1973
2. Schepens CL: Examination of the ora serrata region: Its clinical significance. In Acta, XVI Concilium Ophthalmologicum, Britannia, 1950, Vol 2, pp 1384–1393. London, British Medical Association, 1951
3. Brockhurst RJ, Schepens CL, Okamura ID: Uveitis II. Peripheral uveitis: Clinical description, complications and differential diagnosis. Am J Ophthalmol 49:1257–1266, 1960
4. Brockhurst RJ, Schepens CL, Okamura ID: Uveitis I. Gonioscopy. Am J Ophthalmol 49:1257–1266, 1960
5. Brockhurst RJ, Schepens CL: Uveitis IV. Peripheral uveitis: The complication of retinal detachment. Arch Ophthalmol 80:747–753, 1968
6. Rutnin U, Schepens CL: Fundus appearance in normal eyes. IV. Retinal breaks and other findings. Am J Ophthalmol 64:1063–1078, 1967
7. Dobbie JG: Cryotherapy in the management of toxoplasma retinochoroiditis. Trans Am Acad Ophthalmol Otolaryngol 72:364, 1968
8. Ghartey KN, Brockhurst RJ: Photocoagulation of active toxoplasmic retinochoroiditis. Am J Ophthalmol 89:858, 1980
9. Spalter HF, Campbell CJ, Noyori KS, et al: Prophylactic photocoagulation of recurrent toxoplasmic retinochoroiditis: A preliminary report. Arch Ophthalmol 75:21, 1966
10. Michelson JB, Chisari FV: Behçet's disease: A review. Surv Ophthalmol 26:190, 1982
11. Michelson JB: A Color Atlas of Uveitis Diagnosis. Chicago, Yearbook Medical Publishers, 1984
12. Schepens CL: Retinal Detachment and Allied Diseases, Vol 2. Philadelphia, WB Saunders, 1983

ELEVEN

Intra-ocular Foreign Body With Uveitis or Retinal Detachment

Uveitis with or without retinal detachment may often be a masquerade syndrome for an unsuspected or undetected foreign body that may have traumatized and entered the eye. While this situation may be relatively infrequent in fresh cases of retinal detachment, in cases of patients with smoldering uveitis (Fig. 11-1) the eye may have harbored a foreign body for months, sometimes years, and these cases are often refractory to treatment as the intra-ocular inflammation continues to smolder.

Any eye with a retinal break or a retinal detachment with overlying vitreous inflammation, with or without anterior segment inflammation, may arouse suspicion of harboring intra-ocular foreign body, based either on the patient's history or on clinical signs. Careful assembling of a detailed clinical history and the findings from external examination helps determine the direction the foreign body travels inside the eye. The patient may be wholly unaware that his eye was struck by a foreign body, but careful attention to detail in the history including the tasks of the patient prior to the onset of inflammation in the eye, the patient's occupation, and the patient's hobbies may lead to suspicion of intra-ocular foreign body. Examination of the lids and careful slit lamp inspection of the palpebral and bulbar conjunctiva, sclera, and cornea are performed to look for a suspected perforation site. Gonioscopy should be done in all cases since small foreign bodies are occasionally lodged in the trabecular meshwork where they can be seen inciting an ongoing smoldering uveitis. Before the pupil is dilated, the

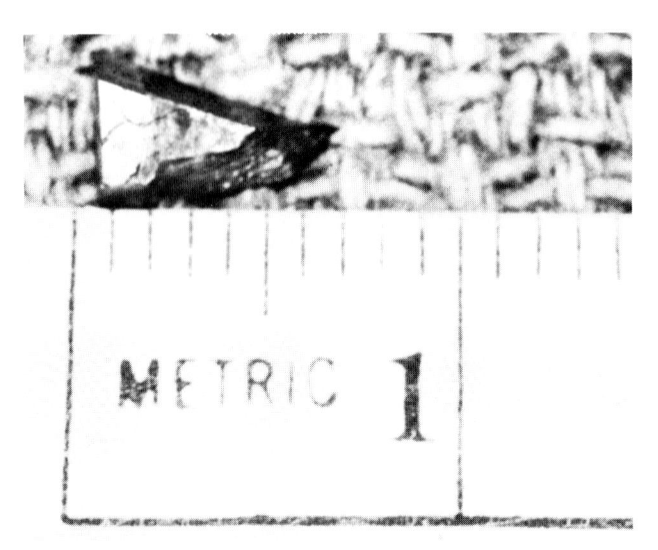

Figure 11-1. Measurement of intra-ocular foreign body removed at vitrectomy from the patient in Figure 11-4 who was unaware of the metallic projectile that had entered the eye, causing a smoldering uveitis.

iris should be scanned for an iris perforation. The lens should be examined for the possibility of a perforation site in its capsule and some cases of lens-induced uveitis may indeed be a masquerade for cases of unsuspected intra-ocular foreign body.

In all cases of intra-ocular foreign body, the danger of subsequent retinal detachment is usually omnipresent. This may occur at any time after the trauma even though no foreign body remains lodged in the eye. A retinal detachment may be noted a few months to many years later, and while it may be suspected that retinal detachment is due to tractional forces from the intra-ocular inflammation, it may, indeed, be the result of a tear or hole in the retina from the foreign body. In such cases the retinal breaks are not always at the site of the original wound; sometimes they are very distant from it, being caused by traction bands that may have developed as a result of the trauma, and may even be found in the posterior pole sometimes as a result of "contra-coupe" forces. Inflammatory bands may be attached to various points of the retina and are often due to connective tissue that grew from the perforation site. Some of these cases, especially in small children, may simulate a *Toxocara canis* infestation. A large band may be seen passing from the perforation site on the surface of the retina to the posterior pole or optic nerve head.

When the presence of an intra-ocular foreign body is suspected in an eye threatened with or already affected by retinal detachment, it is particularly important to perform careful ophthalmoscopy, slit lamp microscopy, radiography and, when particularly useful, both A- and B-scan ultrasonography.

The entrance site of the foreign body that affects the posterior segment of the globe is frequently within the area of the ora serrata and may be visible with the ophthalmoscope as a white scar from which connective tissue fans out into the vitreous cavity. Neovascularization on the retinal surface may occur, and large stalks may bud from the area of rupture up into the vitreous gel. The phenomenon is also seen from the "surgical" perforation site after pars plana vitrectomy. Sometimes a foreign body stops on the wall of the sclera at the entrance site. More often, however, the foreign body is found either in the vitreous cavity or on the opposite side of the eye, even imbedded in the sclera. A foreign body such as a fine metal wire may perforate the globe and not remain inside. Sometimes a foreign body becomes lodged in the orbit after having transfixed the globe in two positions.

Ophthalmoscopy often permits observation of the foreign body and gives an idea of its transparency to light rays in its mobility. Transparent plastic material or glass, with the refractive index close to that of the ocular fluids, may be difficult to see. In such a case radiography may not be useful when the foreign body is radioluscent, but A-scan ultrasound may be of more help than B-scan ultrasound, giving the distinct reflection of an object that is located in the ocular media.

Evaluation of the mobility of the foreign body is important, and it may be advisable to place the patient on a tilting table for this purpose, or having the patient roll gently from side to side utilizing "real time" ultrasound examination. Placing a strong magnet in a suitable location and observing the behavior of the foreign body by ophthalmoscopy will aid in determining its pre-operative degree of magnetism for possible magnetic removal from the eye at the pars plana. However, one must be exceptionally careful in this exploratory phase not to cause excessive movement of a foreign body, thus enabling it to pass into or through structures, causing damage. Sometimes no clear view of the foreign body can be obtained because it is ensheathed in connective tissue or covered in a blanket of hemorrhage inside the eye. Foreign bodies may also become encapsulated in or under the choroid or in the retina itself, forming a retinal granuloma with a foreign body inside. This may then be covered by further scar tissue or an exudate. It is of particular interest that patients who are intravenous drug abusers may be shooting multiple foreign bodies into their retina. Often these are particulate matter of cornstarch, talc, and other diluents of their intravenous drugs that are not filtered out and may even form refractile bodies. These eventually may become encased in granuloma tissue (Figs. 11-2, 11-3).

Usually an encapsulated scar or abscess with surrounding active exudate in the retina or choroid indicates the presence of a reactive foreign body such as steel or brass. The reaction is rarely limited to the area of the foreign body, even when it is encapsulated in the choroid or in the vitreous cavity, but it may cause an extensive intra-ocular reaction, obscuring the etiology of foreign body. There may be extensive exudative choroidal and retinal detachment, inflammatory deposits in the vitreous, on the retina, and on the external surface of the detached retina. Frequently there is spillover of this inflammatory reaction to the anterior

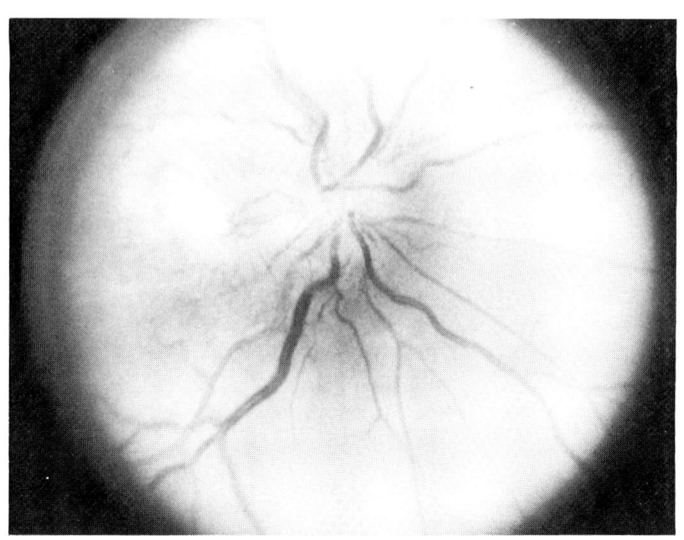

Figure 11-2. A 28-year-old man with encapsulation and abscess formation in the retina of a glistening refractile foreign body, which is now obscured by granuloma formation.

segment that may even simulate a "granulomatous" type of uveitis (Fig. 11-4). The large mutton fat keratic precipitates may be present on the corneal endothelium. The subretinal fluid in such a case is generally thick, viscous, and shifting; the detached retina is usually smooth. A rhegmatogenous retinal detachment may

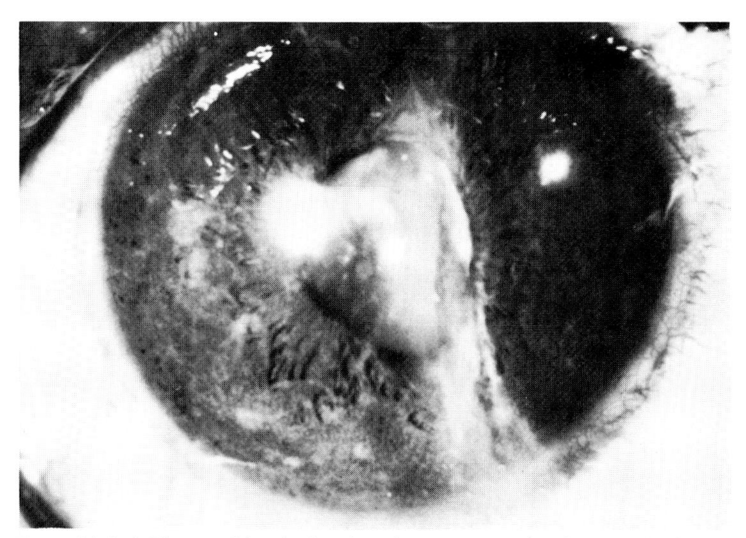

Figure 11-3. A 22-year-old agricultural worker unaware of an intra-ocular foreign body who presented with profound anterior segment inflammation and cataract development with bands of fibrous tissue on the iris surface. The opaque optical media obscured the metallic foreign body lying in the retinal periphery.

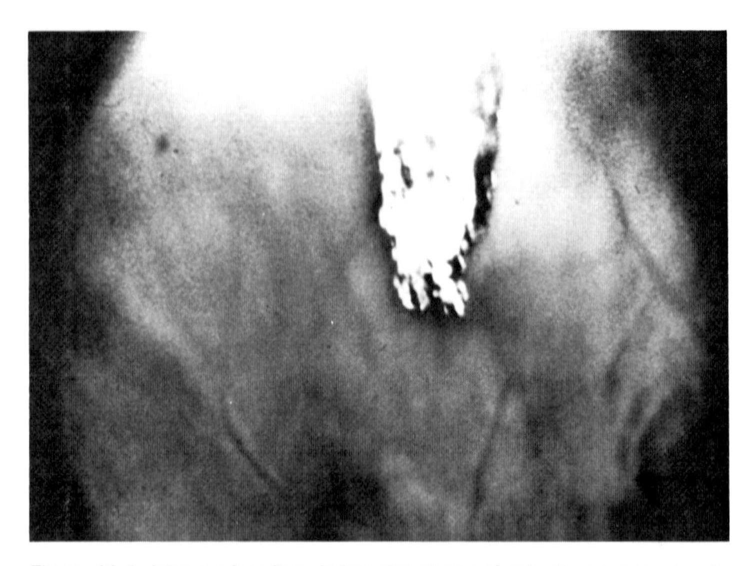

Figure 11-4. Intra-ocular view during vitrectomy of retinal periphery showing large metallic foreign body lying outside of ophthalmoscopic observation, which gave rise to this long-standing case of smoldering uveitis as a mascarade syndrome for a systemic uveitis.

be superimposed on the exudative detachment. By ophthalmoscopy, the vitreous may show fibrous traction bands that often develop in the track of the foreign body inside the vitreous gel. Newly formed tissue may proliferate in the membranes that grow on the back of the retracted vitreous gel and over the retinal surface. These may also grow forward and cover the posterior surface of the lens. The tissue may penetrate the vitreous gel and organize it extensively, later causing multifocal traction retinal detachment, and leading to "massive periretinal proliferation." This latter situation is more likely to occur with large foreign bodies in cases accompanied by a substantial vitreous hemorrhage or following a concurrent subclinical infection in the gel with the foreign body. This is frequently the case when the foreign body material is wood or vegetation and fungal infection is the clinical accompaniment. A careful slit lamp examination of the vitreous changes is indispensable since these alterations are always more extensive than anticipated from ophthalmoscopic examination. Syneresis and vitreous detachment are marked if there has been much inflammatory reaction with the foreign body. In such a case, heavy flare and clumps of cells with cellular debris are seen in the posterior portion of the vitreous. Posterior subcapsular and cortical cataracts often develop at an early stage in this process. These changes may even preclude effective ophthalmoscopic evaluation (Fig. 11-5).

X-ray films or CT scans of the orbit and head should always be taken because they may reveal the presence of several intra-ocular foreign bodies when only one was suspected. If x-ray examination is positive, x-ray localization can be performed. It must be remembered that if the foreign body is intra-ocular, ultrasonography may demonstrate a more precise intra-ocular localization than that

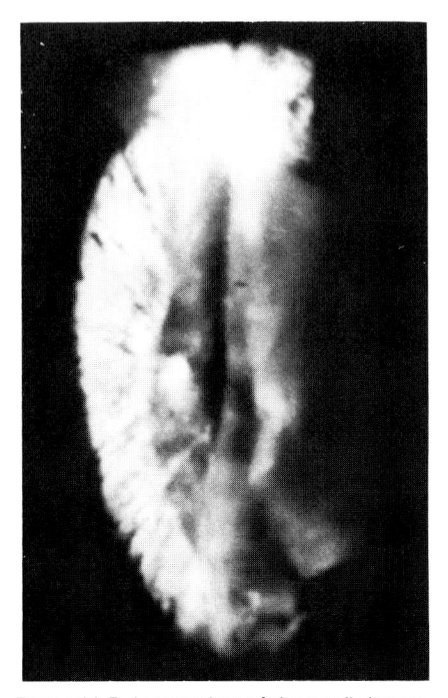

Figure 11-5. Larger view of the pupil demonstrating plastic iritis, fibrous bands on the anterior segment, underlying cataract formation, and dense synechiae of the pupil, which after repeated attempts at dilatation precluded a better ophthalmoscopic view of the back of the eye.

performed by radiography. However, one must remember that the foreign body may be radiolucent or too small to cast a recognizable shadow on radiographic examination.

The ultrasonography, as already alluded to, may be useful in several respects. A-scan helps to locate the foreign body even when it is radiolucent as in the case of glass, plastic, or wood. It also serves to determine the size of the eye. This is important because all methods of x-ray localization are based on the ideal eye size of a 24-mm diameter globe. If the globe is either smaller or larger, the interpretation of x-ray localization may be erroneous. B-scan is useful to give an idea of extent and density of vitreous opacities and the size of retinal detachment that may be obscured and hidden by those opacities and their accompanying hemorrhage.

A copper foreign body inside the globe may be detected as well by ancillary atomic absorptions spectrophotometry. This new technique determines the copper concentration in the aqueous or vitreous fluid and is extremely sensitive with a very low detection level (0.005 micrograms of copper per milliliter). Analysis can be carried out in small samples (0.15–0.35 ml) and can be used for metals other than copper as well.

Siderosis

Two metals, iron and copper, are exceptionally toxic to the eye. The signs these metals elicit inside the eye are pathognomonic for their damage to ocular structures. When these signs are present, even in the absence of a positive history of ocular trauma or the localization or identification of an intra-ocular foreign body, the existence of such an intra-ocular foreign body containing either iron or copper is practically a certainty. The profound nature of the ocular disturbance depends upon the concentration of iron or copper content in the foreign body and its location. Anterior foreign bodies of both copper and iron usually cause more profound changes than posterior ones. Encapsulated or intralenticular foreign bodies usually cause a more chronic and benign but more smoldering reaction, and an anterior segment inflammation of a smoldering nature may obscure the underlying intralenticular foreign body, especially if it is small.

It is essential to remove iron- and copper-containing foreign bodies at an early stage before they produce marked reaction, become encapsulated, or cause total retinal toxicity. Siderosis is more marked with pure steel, which is also more magnetic than alloys of steel such as those used in stainless steel. The iris becomes rust colored and forms posterior synechiae; the pupil can become permanently dilated and paralyzed from it. Open-angle glaucoma frequently results from the smoldering inflammation. The lens may show fine subcapsular rust spots and, indeed, sometimes the whole lens may become yellow. At a later stage large subepithelial rust spots form under the pupillary edge of the lens capsule, and this is usually accompanied by anterior cell and flare, along with cells in the retrolental (Berger's) space. The vitreous contains clouds of rust spots that stick to the degenerated framework of the vitreous gel and zonular fibers. Retinal pigmentary degeneration develops, mostly in the fundus periphery at first, and later progresses toward the macula. The retinal vessels show sclerosis and, later, actual closure. Retinal detachment with or without retinal breaks is common. Retinal toxicity occurs even in the absence of "rust signs" in the retinal pigment epithelium. Electroretinography and electro-oculography may demonstrate the profound visual loss, which is often in excess of the retinal signs of this visual loss.

Chalcosis

Copper or copper alloys often produce a violent reaction in the eye and may cause chalcosis. Copper may, in fact, be the metal most injurious to the eye. When copper is present in the vitreous cavity, dense infiltrates adhere to the retina, usually within a few days of injury. A bluish-green ring forms in the cornea in or near the periphery of Descemet's membrane and represents a traumatic Kayser-Fleisher ring. A typical "sunflower" cataract is produced in the anterior subcapsular layers of the lens, which is said to be pathognomonic of chalcosis. The iris becomes green, and fine metallic particles may be visible in the aqueous on the zonular fibers and on the framework of the syneratic disorganized vitreous gel. Brightly shining copper deposits may be seen in the retina, mostly along the course of the vessels at the posterior pole and in the macula. The electroretinogram is initially markedly depressed, even when little damage is seen inside the eye, and often becomes extinguished early, out of proportion to retinal findings. Therefore, copper-containing foreign bodies must be extracted at the earliest possible stage of their identification and localization. Retinal breaks and retinal detachment accompanying or resulting from intra-ocular foreign bodies should be treated immediately, often concurrent with the removal of the foreign body itself.

Treatment of Retinal Detachment

If retinal breaks are found and the foreign body is no longer inside the eye, a routine scleral buckling may be all that is needed. The extent of buckling is directly related to the degree of vitreous organization as determined by the ophthalmoscopic and slit lamp findings. When vitreous organization is marked, vitreous surgery may have to be considered either at the same time as the scleral buckling or at a separate session, depending on the extent of retinal traction.

If a foreign body and retinal breaks are present, the first decision is whether to remove the foreign body. A nonmagnetic foreign body of relatively small size requires transcleral surgery for removal and should not be extracted unless it is chemically active and causes either an inflammatory reaction, such as has been described, or proliferative reaction in the vitreous cavity. Small fragments of glass or plastic material may be well tolerated in the vitreous. When their presence inside the eye is associated with a rhegmatogenous retinal detachment, the detachment is repaired and the continuing presence of the foreign body seems to cause no further damage. A sizable, chemically inactive intra-ocular foreign body that moves around in the vitreous cavity nearly always causes considerable mechanical irritation, may cause further retinal breaks or tears and formation of vitreous bands and preretinal membranes.

When an intra-ocular foreign body causes an exudative reaction, with or without concomitant retinal breaks, its removal is imperative. A concomitant rhegmatogenous detachment cannot be repaired until the foreign body is removed, owing to the exudative reaction it causes.

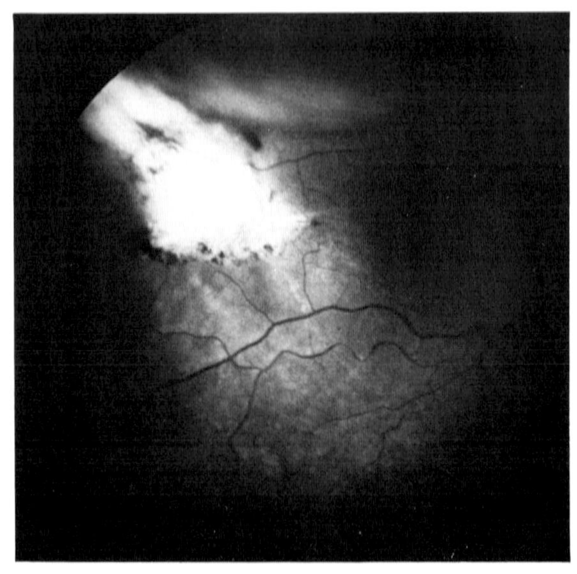

Figure 11-6. Postoperative view of the fundus, cleared by vitrectomy and cataract extraction, demonstrating a hole in the retina from the metallic foreign body situated on the scleral buckle. A contiguous retino-choroidal scar can be seen posterior to it.

Extraction of Foreign Body

Indications for removal of an intra-ocular foreign body vary with the case. Multiple tiny foreign bodies often cannot be removed safely. Nonreactive foreign bodies of small or moderate size are frequently well tolerated. Nonreactive foreign bodies of large size are generally located in the vitreous cavity. As stated above, they move around and cause chronic irritation; therefore, they should be removed. An attempt should also be made to remove foreign bodies that are reactive, whether magnetic or not. Extensive traction bands caused by a long-standing intra-ocular foreign body often produce retinal breaks and retinal detachment and lead to intractable progressive vitreoretinopathy (Fig. 11-6). In such a case newly formed tissue may continue to proliferate as long as the foreign body is present, and its removal should precede retinal detachment surgery.

Four techniques are available to remove intra-ocular foreign bodies.

1. Previous practice was to remove a small, magnetic, easily movable foreign body through the anterior route. This technique is now rarely used, except when a cataract is already present or if an intra-ocular foreign body is lodged in the lens. Other, generally safer, techniques are recommended.

2. The open-sky technique is easiest for the removal of foreign bodies that are either large or multiple, particularly when multiple foreign bodies are encapsulated.
3. Removal through the pars plana is the technique most frequently used. It is indicated for magnetic foreign bodies that are not embedded in the wall of the eye at another location, for all relatively small foreign bodies found in eyes with extensive or total retinal detachment, and for all fairly small nonmagnetic or immovable foreign bodies located in the vitreous and for which extraction is indicated.
4. Removal through the posterior route is indicated for all foreign bodies that are embedded in the wall of the eye, provided their extraction through this route will not damage large choroidal or retinal vessels. Magnetic foreign bodies that are less than 3 mm from the wall of the eye, in an area where the retina is not detached, may be removed by the posterior route when appropriately located.

The technique of foreign body extraction by a transcleral technique, either through the pars plana ciliaris or through the posterior route, is facilitated if the eye is pre-operatively softened to minimize or prevent loss of vitreous. This can be accomplished by a paracentesis or by the use of hypotensive medication such as carbonic anhydrase inhibitors, mannitol, or glycerol.

Movable magnetic foreign body is best extracted through pars plana ciliaris. This generally requires that the foreign body be displaced from another location. As a rule, its maneuverability is best accomplished with a giant magnet prior to surgery, to avoid possible contamination of the surgical field with the magnet. If there is a concomitant retinal detachment, foreign body extraction may be done at the time of retina surgery. If removal is likely to be difficult and the macula is already damaged, it may be preferable to perform the retina surgery 1 to 2 weeks after removal of the foreign body.

The site selected is 4.5 mm from the limbus, in an area in which the epithelium of the pars plana ciliaris is attached, and away from the long ciliary arteries and nerves. As far as possible, the locus should be at the other end of a globe diameter that passes through the location of the foreign body. Such a choice will prevent collision of the foreign body against the retina when it is moved toward the scleral incision. The scleral incision is the same as in pars plana surgery. After exposure of choroid and its treatment by diathermy to prevent hemorrhage, a knuckle of choroid is allowed to prolapse slightly while the sterile tip of an electromagnet is applied directly to this knuckle. One can often appreciate the "pulsation" of the knuckle as the foreign body comes to it. Since only the thin pars plana ciliaris lies between the magnet tip and the foreign body, there is usually no difficulty in pulling the foreign body through this membrane. Most times, a small foreign body will "jump" through the knuckle and onto the electromagnet. In some cases, especially with large or weakly magnetic foreign bodies, it may be necessary to incise the knuckle of pars plana ciliaris with a

Wheeler knife or super blade prior to foreign body removal. Every effort should be made to avoid unnecessary pressure or traction on the globe at this time since an elevation of intra-ocular pressure may result in a large loss of vitreous. If the foreign body lies on retina or is encapsulated in it, the moment of "purchase" by the magnet may cause large retinal tears as the metal spins during its initial polarization by the magnet. There is no way to minimize this complication when the magnet is turned on. Wound closure is performed by pulling up a preplaced mattress suture. The latter may be reinforced by three fine sutures of nonabsorbable material.

If a foreign body is magnetic but encapsulated and rendered immobile by bands or membranes, it must be removed by techniques reserved for nonmagnetic foreign bodies at the pars plana ciliaris. The pars plana ciliaris route is generally advisable except when the foreign body is embedded in the wall of the eye, away from the pars plana ciliaris. However, even in the latter case, if the foreign body lies over a large retinal or choroidal blood vessel, the pars plana route is indicated. When traction bands and membranes are present in the vitreous cavity, they should be removed with a vitrectomy instrument used in conjunction with vitreous forceps. This technique has the additional advantage of providing powerful endo-illumination, which makes vitreous structures more visible.

If a magnetic foreign body is embedded in the wall of the eye or located less than 3 mm from the retina, it may be removed through the posterior route. After exposure of the area of sclera under which the foreign body is located, its position is determined by ophthalmoscopy and transillumination. When the foreign body is in the vitreous cavity, its distance from the retina can be evaluated by the distance between the foreign body and its shadow as seen through the ophthalmoscope.

The procedure for exploration is a scleral undermining, just as one would prepare a scleral bed for a retinal "trapdoor" implant. The area undermined is treated with diathermy or cryoapplications and two mattress sutures of 4-0 polyester (Dacron) are placed on the scleral flaps. Then localization of the foreign body is repeated by ophthalmoscopy and transillumination. If the shadow of the foreign body on the thinned sclera is poorly outlined and the foreign body is 3 mm or more from the choroid, an attempt must be made to bring it in contact with the wall of the eye with a magnet. If this cannot be accomplished, it means that the foreign body is too weakly magnetic, that it is held away from the wall of the eye by tissue proliferation, or that it is encapsulated. In either of these latter cases, it may be better to stop and then to remove the foreign body through the pars plana ciliaris.

If the shadow cast by the foreign body on the undermined sclera is sharp, the undermining should be located so that the foreign body is slightly anterior to its center. A sclerotomy is performed directly over the scleral shadow, and the knuckle of choroid is thoroughly treated with diathermy. A hand magnet is applied to the treated choroid, and the foreign body is removed through the retina and choroid. If the foreign body creates a bulge in the choroid without perforating it, a careful sharp blade incision of the tissue over the knuckle permits completion of the extraction. A previously prepared silicone implant is then inserted under the mattress sutures, which are immediately tied. The hole in the sclera and choroid through which the foreign body was removed should lie on the anterior slope of the segmental buckle. Cryopexy should be applied to the area to enhance chorioretinal adhesion.

When the retina is detached in the area through which the foreign body could be removed, removal should proceed through the pars plana ciliaris, since retinal traction, ripping of the retina, and improper localization, of the foreign body are almost certain to occur.

A large nonmagnetic foreign body may be extracted through the posterior route. This procedure is indicated only when a nonmagnetic foreign body that needs to be removed is embedded in the wall of the eye, is located close to the wall of an eye with attached retina, or is located under detached retina. Pre-operative slit lamp examination of the vitreous cavity with a contact lens or 60 or 90 diopter lens reveals the density of the attachments of the foreign body to exudative or organized material. If the foreign body is surrounded by vitreous gel, there is a chance of removing it easily. If it is surrounded by liquid vitreous in an older patient, a previously vitrectomized patient, or a high myope the chance of successful removal by this technique is slim because the globe will probably collapse before the foreign body is removed. In such a case, the pars plana route should be used. The posterior route of extraction may be indicated if the foreign body is 1 mm or less away from the attached retina. The extraction procedure is similar to that described already: the incision of the undermined sclera must be located accurately over the foreign body. The choroid is incised after its thorough treatment with diathermy. Slight pressure on the globe should force vitreous gel and the foreign body to protrude through the choroidal incision for direct visualization. The foreign body is grasped with forceps and the vitreous gel adherent to it is cut with scissors placed between the foreign body and the globe.

If the foreign body fails to present itself through the gaping choroidal incision, the situation must be evaluated by ophthalmoscopy and transillumination. The incision may be too small or slightly misplaced. If too small, the incision is carefully enlarged. If misplaced, the linear incision may be transformed into a T-shaped or L-shaped one. This may require enlargement of the scleral bed. If ophthalmoscopy reveals that slight pressure on the globe does not push the foreign body into the choroidal incision, the foreign body is probably too far inside the vitreous cavity for this technique to be used. An attempt must then be made to extract the foreign body with vitreous forceps, generally through the pars plana ciliaris after closure of the posterior incision. The turgor of the globe must be re-established before moving on to the pars plana approach. Removal of almost all nonmagnetic foreign bodies that are in liquid vitreous, or in front of a large intra-ocular vessel, or ensheathed in connective tissue, or more than 1 mm from the retina must be performed through the pars plana ciliaris as already described.

If a foreign body is known to be present but cannot be seen by ophthalmoscopy because of opacities in the media, it is essential to localize it beforehand. A study by B-scan ultrasonography will indicate whether the retina is attached or detached and the probable relation of the retina, and other membranes, to the foreign body. It should be remembered, however, that ultrasound is not a very reliable technique for localizing intra-ocular foreign bodies. Even with opaque media, a foreign body often will cast a shadow on the sclera by transillumination, if it is located close to the sclera. In this type of case it should be noted that the accuracy of transillumination augments those supplied by other instruments that use the principle of electrical induction, such as the Berman or Bronson locator.

In most instances in which the vitreous is opaque, foreign body removal should not be undertaken until the vitreous has been cleared by vitrectomy. If the foreign body is small and either immobile or nonmagnetic, it should be extracted by a two-instrument technique using vitreous forceps and the vitrectomy tip. If it is mobile and magnetic, it is removed with a magnet through the pars plana incision after carefully cutting, incising, and nibbling the vitreous opacities. "Open sky" vitrectomy may be the only alternative for cases of large foreign bodies in order to maintain the integrity of ocular tissues and structures.

References

1. Bronson NR: II: Management of magnetic foreign bodies. In Freeman HM (ed): Ocular Trauma, pp 179–186. New York, Appleton-Century-Crofts, 1979
2. Coleman DJ: Ultrasonic evaluation of the vitreous. In Freeman HM, Hirose T, Schepens CL (eds): Vitreous Surgery and Advances in Fundus Diagnosis and Treatment, pp 63–77. New York, Appleton-Century-Crofts, 1977
3. Rosenthal AR, Hopkins JL, Appleton B et al: Studies on intraocular copper foreign bodies: Atomic absorption spectrophotometry. Arch Ophthalmol 92:431–436, 1974
4. Duke-Elder S, MacFaul PA: System of Ophthalmology. Vol XIV. Injuries. Part I. Mechanical Injuries, pp 515–523, 525–542, 579–611. London, Henry Kimpton, 1972
5. Neubauer H: Management of nonmagnetic intraocular foreign bodies. In Freeman HM (ed): Ocular Trauma, pp 187–196. New York, Appleton-Century-Crofts, 1979
6. Harris D, Brockhurst RJ: Localization of intraocular foreign bodies by transillumination, and by indirect ophthalmoscopy with scleral indentation. Can Med Assoc J 87:565–567, 1962
7. Leopold P: Reperage des corps etrangers intra-oculaires par la diaphanoscopie transpupillaire. Ann Oculist 192:863–867, 1959
8. Minsky H: Transscleral removal of intraocular foreign body with the aid of the Berman locator. Arch Ophthalmol 31:207–210, 1944
9. Schepens CL: Retinal Detachment and Allied Diseases, Vol 2. Philadelphia, WB Saunders, 1983

TWELVE

Laser Surgery for Ocular Inflammatory Disease

Light energy has been used in the treatment of various ocular disorders and problems for more than 40 years. Dr. Gerd Meyer-Schwickerath developed the first laser device to focus fine rays of the sun into a beam that could be directed into the eye of a patient to photocoagulate his retina. Thus began the era of laser treatment for ocular disorders, and more widely for the rest of medicine in general. Dr. Schwickerath obtained this idea from patients who received retinal burns from viewing an eclipse of the sun. As a result of his early treatments, a xenon arc lamp photocoagulator was developed in 1950 and was the first to be used to treat vascular problems and tumors of the choroid and retina. Further advances in technology in the 1960s saw the precise harnessing of various wavelengths of light. The laser, an acronym for Light Amplification by the Stimulated Emission of Radiation, is an electro-optical device capable of transmitting an intense beam of light energy. Each laser has three basic components: (1) a lasing medium that can be a gas, liquid or solid; (2) an excitation source that will pump high energy into the medium; and, (3) a resonator, which is a chamber consisting of two parallel mirrors, one of them totally reflective and the other partially reflective.

The principle of laser beam operation is simple. When the coherent atoms drop from a higher to a lower energy state they release energy in the form of photons. The wavelength of the emitted photons is a function of the difference between the two energy levels. In the laser, many atoms are poised in a high energy state ready to be dropped to a lower one. These high energy atoms will spontaneously emit photons of energy. When one photon strikes another high energy atom, it causes another photon of identical wavelength to be emitted traveling in the same direction. As these photons are released and phased with one another, the light wave becomes a multiple of the original intensity. Each of these released photons can then cause the stimulated emission of additional photons and additional energy. In the laser this wave passes back and forth many times between mirrors, becoming amplified, sweeping more photons with it in a beam that increases rapidly along the longitudinal axis of the chamber. A portion of this light is allowed to leak out through the partially reflective mirror constituting the active emission from the laser, hence the laser beam which is used for treatment.

There are three basic aspects of laser energy that differentiate it from ordinary lamplight or sunlight.

1. It is monochromatic and releases energy at just one or a few very discreet wave lengths.
2. It is coherent. The waves or emitted photon energy of the laser light are all on the same phase. Monochromatic light produced by any means other than a laser has phase differences between the waves.
3. Collimation. The beam of laser-emitted energy remains almost perfectly parallel along its path with minimal loss of power due to divergence.

Of the many types of industrial and experimental lasers being developed today, only four are commonly used in general surgery and ophthalmology. These include the carbon dioxide laser, the argon laser, the krypton laser, and the neodymium-yttrium aluminum garnet (Nd:YAG) laser (Fig. 12-1). The latter three are the most commonly used lasers in practice today. Some carbon dioxide lasers are in use for intra-ocular photocoagulation during surgery. In general, the argon laser and krypton laser are used to photocoagulate the retina and choroid and "burn" it, sealing tissue. The YAG laser and most current carbon dioxide lasers are used for cutting purposes.

Many factors combine to determine the nature and extent of the thermal effect of lasers: the power density or energy density, the spot size, and the nature of the light interaction with the tissue. The total power output of the laser is measured in watts. The thermal effect induced in target tissues is a function of the power density (W/cm^2) and the energy density measured as power density multiplied by time indicates a total amount of energy or radiation to a given tissue area. The spot size and measure of the surface area in which the laser light is directed is an important concept. Spot size is an important determining factor of power density because density varies as the inverse of the area. At a constant power, power density increases by reducing the spot size. The ability to regulate the laser spot size depends upon the wavelength, the means of delivery, and the focusing of a particular laser.

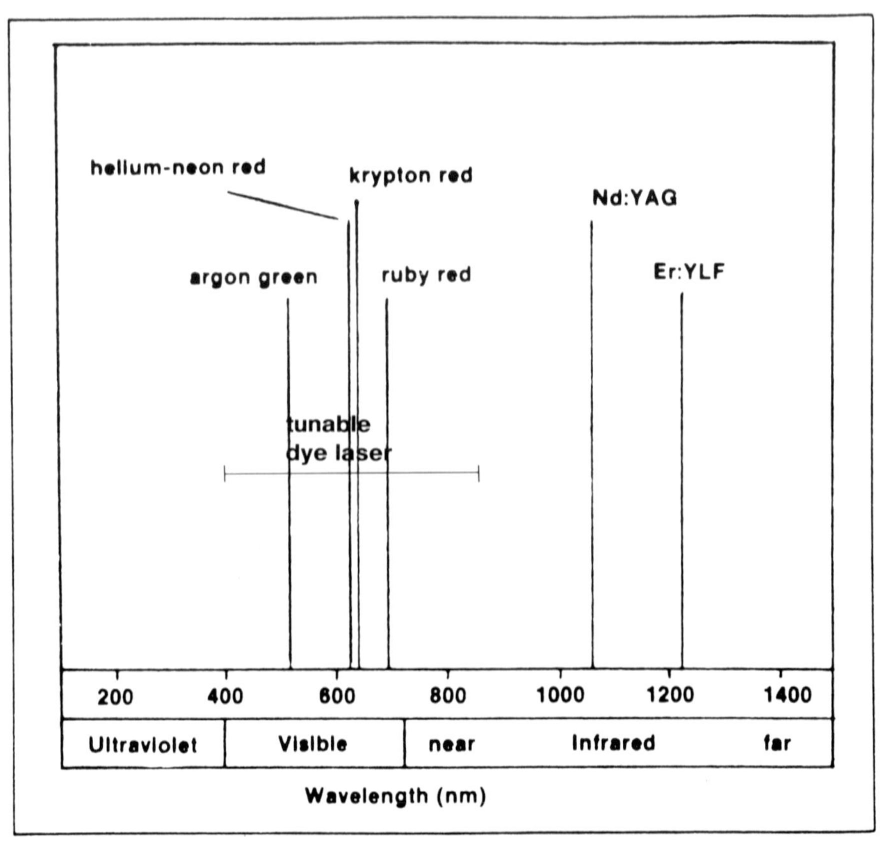

Figure 12-1. Wavelength emissions of various ophthalmic lasers.

While the krypton and argon laser do find applications in cases of intra-ocular inflammation when retinal tear formation and retinal hole formation occur, perhaps the most boldly theoretical laser for use in ocular inflammatory disease will be the Nd:YAG laser. It will allow us to lyse tissues in the eye, thereby enabling us to disrupt synechiae, inflammatory bands, and fibrous traction bands in the front and, more important, in the back of the eye. However, one must not gloss over the usefulness of the former two lasers. Most important, retinal tears and retinal holes still need to be sealed in some instances by an argon laser. This is its primary application in this disease category. The krypton laser, although it has been used to extirpate subretinal neovascular membranes and because it has unique light-absorbing capacities that would render it absorbed more readily in the retinal pigment epithelium and in the choroid than in the inner retinal layers (thereby sparing them), has found more use in its ability to seal holes or tears or to perform photocoagulation in the diabetic state. The krypton laser is also employed in patients with a hemorrhage in the vitreous or even in the anterior segment, or with inflammation in the vitreous with pigmented cells that would prevent the absorption of argon laser to the area of the retina that needs application. Thus, the krypton has also been employed in patients with both intra-ocular inflammatory disease and diabetes for retinal applications since the argon laser, which would have been used otherwise, would have its energy application absorbed and dissipated into the cells and material in the vitreous.

Both the argon laser and the YAG laser have been used also for the treatment of glaucoma. However, in most inflammatory states, treatment of the glaucoma must still remain surgical. It is the inflammation that is usually causative of the glaucoma, and eyes that are inflamed are not appropriate candidates for laser trabeculoplasty, which has even more short-term results than surgical trabeculectomy in such a situation.

The YAG laser holds the most promise in the treatment of intra-ocular inflammatory disease where conventional surgery was used previously. YAG lasers were first built for industrial and military applications for warfare. The output powers were too low to produce optical breakdown in the eye. Only after development of lasers capable of emitting high power through very short pulses did the possibility of using optical radiation in the production of "plasma" become a viable method for ophthalmological treatment. Early ruby crystal lasers were used to treat retinal disorders, but when experimentally applied to the lens capsule, they were inadequate in rupturing the transparent capsular bag. Krasnoff performed experiments in the 1970s that proved that high peak power pulses could be used clinically to produce ocular disruption. He then incorporated the Q-switched ruby laser in the treatment of open-angle glaucoma. Unable to rupture the lens capsule in human eyes with a senile cataract, Krasnoff developed a technique for transferring iris pigment deposits onto the capsule to facilitate absorption of the ruby light energy leading to rupture of the capsule.[1]

Nobel laureates Dausset and Bessis demonstrated in the 1970s that obliteration of a mitochondrial body within a blood cell could be performed by a pulsed YAG laser. During this time Aron-Rosa[2] used mode-locking to obtain high-power pulses, thus creating plasma shock waves, which she applied to vitreous membranes while Fankhauser and his colleagues[3] used Q-switching to achieve high-powering YAG laser application for treatment of glaucoma (Fig. 12-2). Lasers with continuous-wave output and laser-pulsed output have been used in ophthalmology (Fig. 12-3). The continuous-wave lasers as already noted (argon, krypton) are used to produce heat and coagulation by absorption of light in the tissues, thereby causing a burn.[4] Even though these lasers are considered to be of low total output, they can have beam intensities far in excess of the most powerful lights per unit of power because they have minimal angular divergence of their energy beams.[5] The pulsed laser emission that persists for a nanosecond (10^{-9}) or picosecond (10^{-12}) achieves tissue disruption by focusing its energy to create high-powered density in a small target area. Because this effect has a threshold, it is called nonlinear and requires a minimum power concentration. When the light threshold is achieved, ionization of matter occurs with production of pressure waves through tissue (a mini "explosion" phenomenon). Damage to tissue is

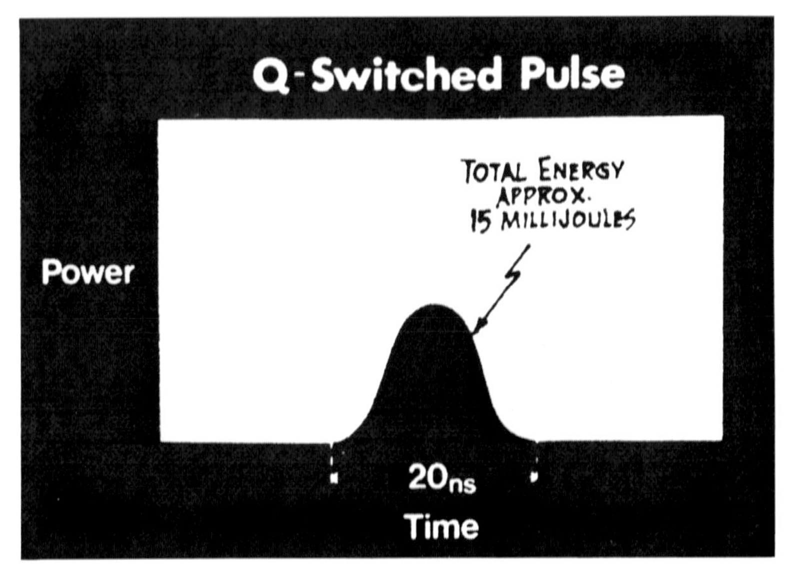

Figure 12-2. This graph depicts the power delivery over time of a Q-switched pulse of laser energy.

caused by decompensation of the ionization and shock waves rather than by tissue coagulation due to heat as noted in the argon and krypton lasers.[6]

The Nd:YAG laser employs the medium of neodymium diffused into an yttrium aluminum garnet crystal. When this is fashioned into a cylindrical rod and illuminated by a xenon flash tube discharge, the neodymium atoms absorb energy and create the necessary population of excitable atoms that give rise to laser action and energy discharge. The main output of the Nd:YAG laser is at 1064 nm, which is in the near infrared range in a region where the cornea and lens are both mostly transparent. Since the YAG laser beam is invisible, a red helium/neon (hene) laser beam (632 nm) coincident to the YAG is used for aiming only. This is the small red dot we see focused on the tissues when applying the mode lock or the Q-switch laser. The use of filters in the oculars of the slit lamp protects the operator against backward reflection. The maximum radiation received by the operator falls well under the safety level by a factor of 10^{-6}.

The actual function of a YAG laser is to produce a highly concentrated focus of electromagnetic energy that results in breakdown of the structures in the optical medium. Such a breakdown in a very tiny volume generates a micro "explosion" or shock wave and is called optical breakdown. This occurs when the radiation is of sufficient strength to tear electrons away from the atoms in which it is focused, creating a "plasma" of ionized gas. Since the laser focuses on a microscopic region in space, the resulting destruction is very limited in scope, and may be used to destroy very tiny tissue masses ripping them with the coincident explosion at their surface.

Materials such as blood and water are transparent to the infrared light photons of the Nd:YAG laser, and tissue may be opaque to the visible light spectrum but transparent to certain other wavelengths. Rapid expansion of the nearby region coincident to the laser application also causes an acoustic "crackle" plainly audible to the observer and the patient. In fact when one uses the YAG laser, the visible and the audible effects of the optical breakdown are like a mini "lightening bolt and accompanying thunderstorms" scaled down to our own microscopic slit lamp world in size. The important concept is that no absorption by an opaque medium is required. The action occurs wherever the laser's focal spot is placed in the "mini explosion," and the threshold for optical breakdown is reached. Should there be a membrane or a fibrous band in that region of the posterior capsule, localized mechanical damage can occur and produce a small hole, tear, or rip in the structure. This is the basic principle of surgery with the YAG laser.

The temperature within the area of optical breakdown may exceed 10,000°C, but it is localized on a microscopic level and of such short duration that it is not a dominating feature of the observed tissue interaction and breakdown. The size of the spark of optical breakdown is 0.5 to 0.7 mm. An energy deposit of 1 millijoule induces a shock pressure equal to 10^7 mm Hg during 2×10^{-9} seconds at a distance of 0.1 mm with a power density in the range of $1.5–8 \times 10^{12}$ W/cm^2.[6]

Professor Aron-Rosa states that if the eyeball is considered as a sphere 20 mm in diameter, the pressure wave at the sclera 10 mm away will be 10 mm Hg

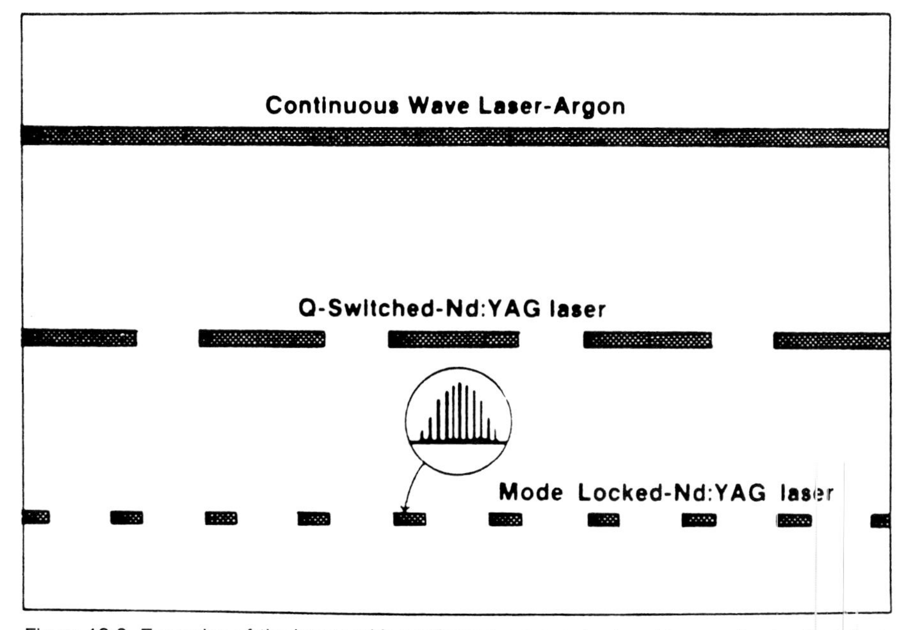

Figure 12-3. Examples of the lasers with continuous-wave output and laser-pulsed output that are used in ophthalmology.

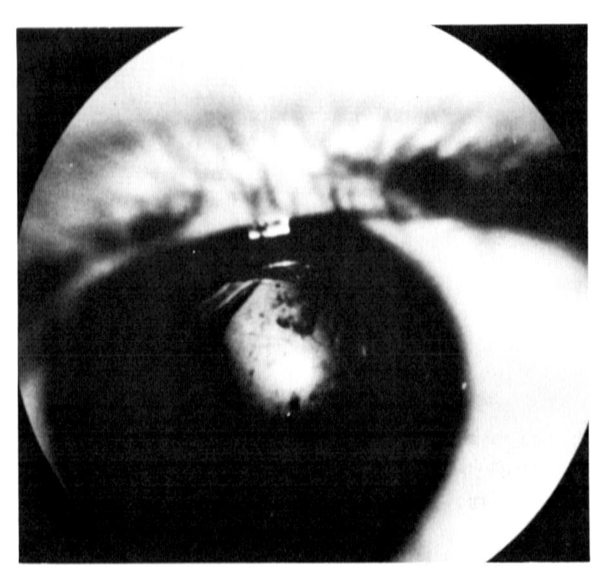

Figure 12-4. Iritis patient with thickened posterior capsule and posterior chamber lens implant.

and decreasing as the inverse to distance during 2×10^{-9} seconds, which should not be harmful to ocular structures as we understand it. The acoustic pressure wave in the "plasma" also contributes to the scatter of pulsed laser light. This is known as the Brillouin scattering. Stimulated Brillouin scattering is produced by the laser beam itself, resulting in a pressure pulse. Neither of these foregoing properties are thought to contribute to ocular damage. However, one must consider what risks might be present in creating laser-induced lesions in the retina and choroid when treating the posterior lens capsule or fibrous bands in the posterior cavity of the eye (Figs. 12-4, 12-5, 12-6). When working in the anterior segment and in front of the posterior capsule, it is felt that any damage to the retina and choroid might be minimal. However, an Nd:YAG laser beam focuses 17 to 20 mm from the pars plana to the retina and should be well diverged before it reaches the retina. Beam diversion is the most important consideration in terms of retinal protection when working in the anterior segment. Plasma formation also protects retinal tissue from damaging radiant energy by absorbing and scattering incident radiation before it reaches the retina.[7-9] However, as the laser burst is focused nearer to the retina, when working on fibrous bands in the vitreous cavity for example, damage is caused by shock waves but not by radiant energy.[7,10,15] Therefore, as we begin to treat vitreous pathology in terms of fibrous bands and vitreous opacities closer to the retina, secondary damage from the shock waves becomes increasingly important.

Early research focused on the question of whether YAG laser bursts could cause rhegmatogenous retinal detachment. In laboratory applications to create experimental YAG lesions in rabbits and other animals, chorioretinal damage

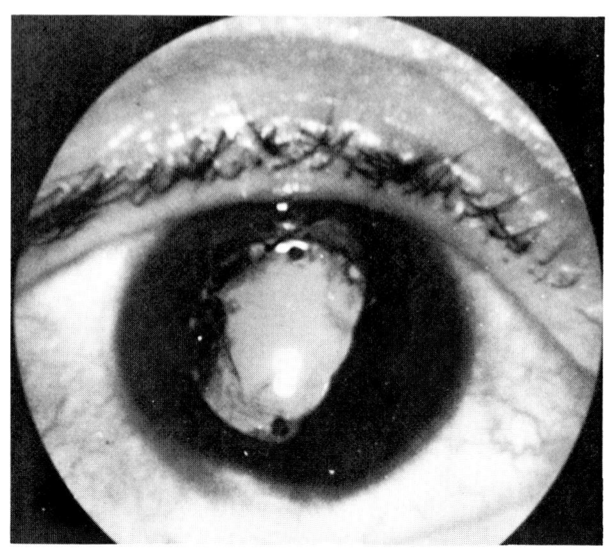

Figure 12-5. Same patient as in Figure 12-4 after YAG capsulotomy.

could be demonstrated. But this damage did not lead to rhegmatogenous retinal detachment. Brown and Benson[14] used the pulsed Nd:YAG laser to treat three patients with persistent diabetic traction retinal detachments. They cut vitreous bands at 3 to 4 mm from the retinal surface and caused the traction to decrease or

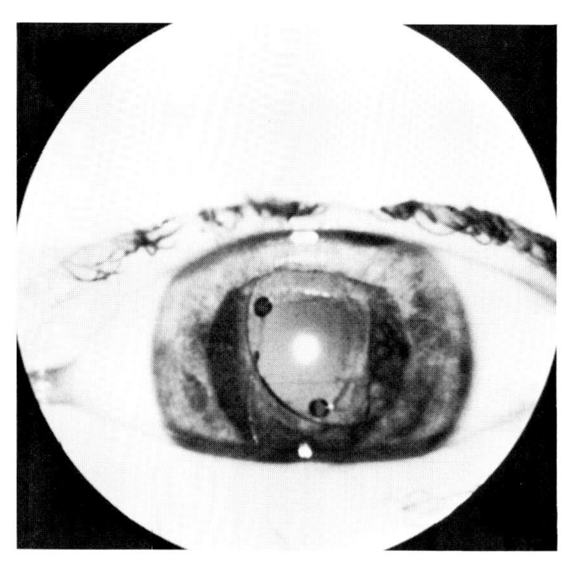

Figure 12-6. Another patient, after extracapsular cataract surgery and posterior chamber lens, with grossly thickened and fibrosed posterior capsule, opened with YAG procedure.

resolve in these three patients. The only complication observed was one choroidal hemorrhage nasal to the disc without visual sequelae. Puliafito[12] treated experimental vitreous membranes in rabbit eyes with a Q-switched Nd:YAG laser. Avascular membranes were cut at 4 mm from the retinal surface, and it was documented that no clinical photographic or fluorescein angiographic evidence of retinal or choroidal damage occurred. Cutting membranes 1.5 to 3 mm from the retinal surface did cause choroidal hemorrhage in four of seven cases. One eye suffered a nonhemorrhagic lesion from laser lysis of the membrane 2 mm in front of the retina. Peyman[18] observed a significant decrease in the threshold energy density needed to create retinal lesions as the pulse duration of the laser was decreased. Thermal energy in close proximity to the retina can also be a factor in producing retinal lesions because it decreases as a square function rather than a cubed function as does acoustical energy. Choroidal hemorrhage may be an indication that Bruch's membrane has been disrupted, increasing the risk of developing subretinal neovascularization, vitreous hemorrhage or both. Manning and colleagues[19] have presented the clinical and histopathological findings of YAG laser lesions in the human eye, from experimental macular injury to the effects of direct YAG laser injury to normal retina.

Q-switching and Mode Locking YAG Laser

Q-switching and mode locking are the techniques employed for pulsing the laser to regulate power density. The ability to pulse a laser provides equivocal needs. In lasers such as the ruby or YAG laser, the medium is pumped to create optical excitation with a flash lamp. These are the high-powered densities that are achieved to produce optical breakdown, and it is necessary to create them with very short bursts of pulsed high power.

There are distinct differences between mode locked and Q-switched YAG lasers (see Fig. 12-3). Mode locked lasers are dependent on a dye system that may bleach unevenly and result in an irregular output of energy. These lasers require relatively long cavities within them to generate longitudinal modes. The flexibility in terms of power adjustment is limited in the mode locked laser, which is controlled by the use of filters. Therefore, these lasers require more space and maintenance and seem to deliver less reproducible energy output with a decreased range of power than the Q-switched laser. The Q-switched laser, on the other hand, may be built with a shorter cavity of less than a half-meter and newer models are even shorter. The shutter device may be a dye or an electrical optical mechanism. The latter is quite reliable and requires little maintenance. These laser systems also have a higher power output than do their mode locked counterparts and may be more useful for dense membranes where obviously a higher power output is necessary. One must remember that there is a difference between the Q-switched and mode locked lasers in time elapsed during pulses (see Fig. 12-3). The pulse width of a mode locked laser is 1/1000 that of a Q-switched laser for a great power density. To produce optical breakdown, therefore, Q-switched lasers require higher energy levels than do mode locked lasers. In the Q-switched laser, one must remember that energy buildup is gradual and the heating of impurities at the focal point contributes to optical breakdown through thermal effects. This is opposite to what happens with a mode locked laser, where the enormous irradiance will cause instantaneous ionization not independent of impurities at the focal site. Hence, optical breakdown is more constant, reliable and predictable, and less explosive with the mode locked laser. However, the Q-switched laser is more suitable for the rupture of strong and thick membranes.

Surgical Applications

The introduction of the pulsed laser to produce optical breakdown, thereby achieving a clean surgical incision, is a major breakthrough in ophthalmic surgery. No "knife" is necessary, no pain is sustained by the patient, and a short slit lamp session supplants a surgical procedure and hospital stay. Most important, in all the possible cutting techniques using a pulsed laser in the eye, the risk of postoperative endophthalmitis from intervention is abolished. It is also possible that the incidence of postoperative complications, such as retinal detachment, retinal tears, and disruption of other ocular structures, will be less frequent in the future because of the possibilities of laser surgery than with surgical procedures by instruments.

So far, the primary employment of the Nd:YAG laser has been for the dicission of membranes in aphakic or pseudophakic patients following cataract extraction. The procedure is straightforward and well tolerated by the patients, producing almost no pain. Depending upon the thickness of the membrane and its surface tension and folds, as few as three or four laser bursts may be all that is necessary to lyse such a capsule when one employs its own surface tension as an aid in selecting where the laser bursts should be placed, allowing for traction forces to further rip and open the capsule. Sometimes as many as several hundred are required to break through an optically dense, thickened, and very fibrous capsule. This same spectrum of energy employment applies equally to posterior capsules, synechiae, the anterior vitreous face when this clouds over in uveitis patients, and fibrous bands in the vitreous cavity, as well. The latter usually require much more energy and many more laser bursts than any of the other preceding fibrous or scarred structures. With regard to distance, the intra-ocular lenses, anterior chamber, or iris supported lenses usually produce no problems because of the greater distance from the posterior capsule. These usually do not form synechiae from the iris to the anterior portion of the implant, as well.

Posterior chamber intra-ocular lenses produce challenges in many respects. The first is the surgeon's focusing skills. The laser beam is usually coaxial and the position of optical breakdown with plasma formation should be deeper than the position of the posterior capsule itself. The front shock wave is employed to open

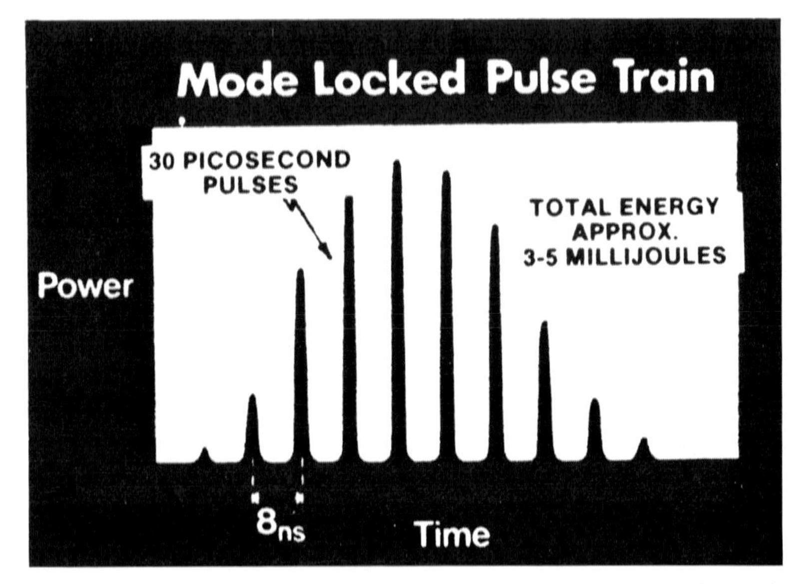

Figure 12-7. This graph demonstrates power in the individual pulses of a mode locked laser and shows the difference in its pulse beats versus the continuous pulse of energy as generated in the Q-switched laser.

the posterior capsule, and this is accomplished by setting the oculars of the eyepiece to +1.00 diopters to move the focal spot back, assuming a better safety position for the posterior chamber lens. The newer posterior chamber lenses address this problem by their design: they are now produced with ridges and structures that yield a larger separation from the capsule.

When a mode locked YAG laser is used for posterior capsulectomy behind a posterior chamber lens, the energy output should usually be in the range of 1 to 3 mJ and often it is necessary to boost this up to 3 to 5 mJ (Fig 12-7). Contact lenses may be useful to maintain a tight focal spot. A +60 diopter Abraham lens can be used to minimize the risk of highly concentrated laser beam striking the lens and to allow better focus ability. Interestingly, the fracture and pitting of posterior chamber lens implants have been seen to range from 80% of eyes with posterior chamber lenses to 20% of cases in a recent FDA report. The highest incidence is usually related to posterior chamber lenses. Also, it is important to remember that no deleterious effects have been reported as a consequence of the release of monomers or of ultraviolet absorbing materials from lenses.[7] There have been only anecdotal reports in the literature of lenses actually fracturing from YAG laser use. When an intra-ocular lens is struck by the YAG laser, there is often minor pitting. Careful focusing and the use of low energy pulses decrease the incidence of lens damage.

Differences do exist among the various types of intra-ocular lenses in regard to their composition, purity, and hardness in their reaction to laser damage. Energy levels of 10 mJ or greater used on injection-molded PMMA lenses have shown 100% cell toxicity. No cytotoxic effect was seen at energy levels of 2 to 5 mJ. The usual power setting one must remember for clinical YAG laser capsulotomy is in the range of 1 to 2 mJ. This is also true of synechiae and anterior segment bands. When one focuses in the vitreous cavity and boosts the power up to 3 to 5 mJ and even higher, one is so posterior to the posterior chamber lens in many of these cases that damage to the lens in this setting should be nonexistent. So far, no apparent difference in toxicity of leachable substance has been demonstrated among the various types of absorptive ultraviolet material used in the intra-ocular lenses and reports state that pitting of the lens has not caused visual problems.[8] Although theoretically glare could result, some newer glass intra-ocular lenses struck by the laser beam have cracked in patients' eyes and the FDA has issued strict warnings advising against photodisruption in the presence of glass lenses. Aiming of the laser perpendicular to the tension lines of the posterior capsule may reduce substantially the number of laser applications because this technique utilizes the innate opening capacity of the capsule itself under tension and stress.

Adhesions and Synechiae

The cutting of adhesions to the lens and to other structures in the anterior segment is also possible with the YAG laser. Theoretically lysis of vitreous bands to the wound may ameliorate or even eliminate cystoid macular edema of a "vitreous wick" syndrome. If vitreous bands are present in excess of 1 or 2 clock hours and are thick and cannot be immediately lysed in the 3 to 5 mJ range, a mechanical vitrectomy is probably a better alternative, since use of the YAG laser may involve excessive energy[9] and may presumably result in rhegmatogenous retinal detachment (the "working area" not being far from the vitreous base), a secondary glaucoma from energy input into the eye, or both. With the aid of a mirror, it is often best to cut a strand in the vitreous at an angle because there is less material and, therefore, fewer laser applications are necessary.[10] Vitreous bands, which then are only partially sectioned and do not float freely, are enabled to maintain a tension in the eye to be cut further. One must plan a strategy for cutting vitreous bands before one proceeds to lyse them in a haphazard fashion. One must be careful when working in the vitreous cavity to focus the beam in a manner that avoids rupture of either the posterior capsule or the anterior hyaloid face if both are present and intact. Rupture of the anterior hyaloid face may cause forward movement of the vitreous, which could cause pupillary block or increase the risk of cystoid macular edema because of movement of vitreous forward into the anterior segment. YAG lasers are currently under investigation for use in cutting vascular membranes in the posterior segment of the eye, and this procedure should not be carried out casually by the cataract surgeon, but is better employed by the retina-vitreous surgeon who is familiar with the mechanisms and relationships in the posterior of the eye.[14]

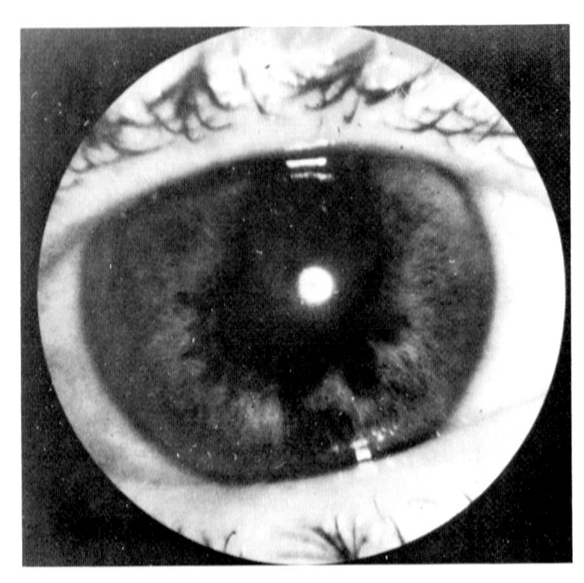

Figure 12-8. Prelaser photograph showing a pupillary block glaucoma in a pseudophakic patient with heavy thickened fibrous synechiae for 180° from 3:00 position down inferiorly all around to the 9:00 position. The synechiae were later lysed using the YAG laser, being careful to avoid the posterior chamber lens.

Patients with uveitis, in whom a posterior chamber lens has been placed, may develop thickening of the anterior hyaloid face even after capsulotomy in that situation. Capsulotomy should be deferred until true optical blurring occurs, because of the purported relationship of cystoid edema to aphakia or pseudoaphakia and a nonintact posterior capsule. Nevertheless, the anterior hyaloid in these uveitis patients may thicken and opacify rather rapidly because of postsurgical intra-ocular inflammation. Many patients have been seen who required laser rupture of an anterior hyaloid that had become as thickened as the posterior capsule had been previously (Fig. 12-8). In several patients, successive lysis or rupture of the hyaloid face was necessary to achieve continuous optical clarity in the presence of ongoing intra-ocular inflammation. In Figure 12-9, this had to be done nine times in order for the patient to maintain vision in the 20/40 to 20/30 range. Each time the patient's anterior hyaloid thickened secondary to intra-ocular inflammation, and the anterior hyaloid resembled the original posterior capsule lysed previously. Such patients, hopefully, may never develop cystoid macular edema even though the hyaloid is opened and may move forward. If this is to occur, the relationship might be due to the open capsule at the open hyaloid face or to the endogenous intra-ocular inflammation alone.

Synechiae may be lysed in the pseudophakic, aphakic, or phakic patients. Of course, the least complications occur in the pseudophakic patient with a poste-

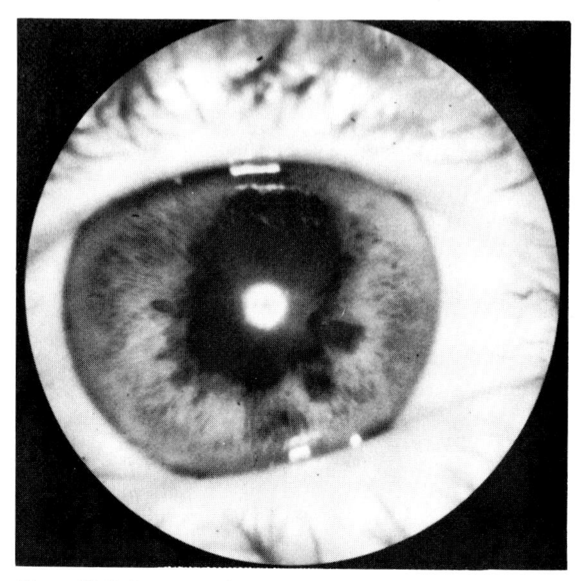

Figure 12-9. Postoperative photograph showing a clear cornea after this pseudophakic-pupillary block glaucoma was relieved by lysing the heavy thickened fibrous synechiae from the 3:00 position down around to the 9:00 position on the posterior chamber lens implant. The pressure was reduced from the 50s down to 18, and aqueous flow was once again re-established.

rior chamber lens. However, even in the phakic patient, synechiolysis has been performed safely with the surgeon being mindful to stay very anterior to the lens capsule, right at the border of the iris cuff or collarette (Fig. 12-10). Laser lysis of such synechiae in an inflamed eye may, in fact, worsen the intra-ocular inflammation due either to iris damage and disruption or to the mechanism of phakolytic glaucoma in which the anterior lens capsule is accidentally ruptured and cortical proteins leak out, thus sensitizing the patient further and worsening his underlying uveitis. Aphakic patients with uveitis can often form pupillary block due to synechiae to the thickened hyaloid, and in such a situation the anterior hyaloid face is better ruptured with a few bursts of YAG laser than with attempts at synechiolysis. While this may release vitreous into the anterior segment and theoretically does increase the risk for cystoid macular edema or even further pupillary block due to hyaloid contiguity, nevertheless, in this one clinical setting, rupture of the hyaloid is preferred to an extensive synechiolysis, which may cause more iris damage and pigment release.

Significant progress has been made using the YAG laser to lyse vitreous wick membranes to cataract incisions. While this was formerly the ken of the vitreous surgeon when limited vitrectomy was thought to reduce the resultant cystoid macular edema from a vitreous wick syndrome, this can be achieved much more safely with a slit lamp session with YAG membrane lysis. Adequate visualization

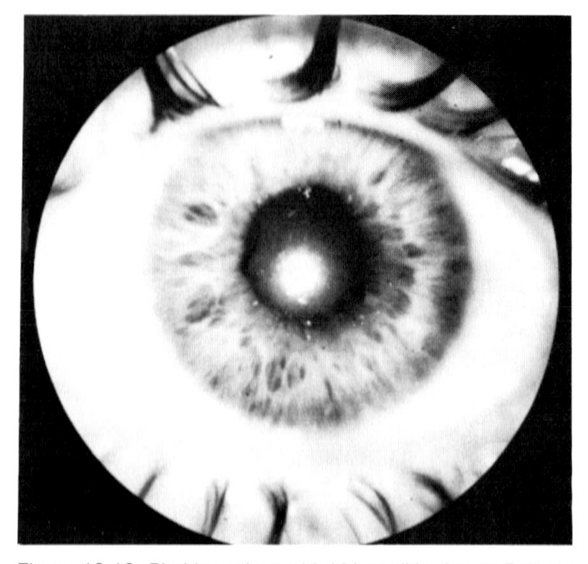

Figure 12-10. Phakic patient with iridocyclitis due to Reiter's disease with bound-down 360° synechiaed pupil with a pupillary block glaucoma. Note the heavy fibrous brown synechiae between the 9:00 and the 12:00 positions. These were later lysed close to the iris collarette, being careful to avoid the anterior lens capsule, which relieved the pupillary block glaucoma and averted an intraocular surgery for this patient using the YAG laser.

of all vitreous wick bands to the cataract wound is central to the achievement of success in this procedure. Often it is difficult to visualize all of these and extensive laser applications are needed in that area of the original cataract wound closure. Where there is structural deformity of the pupil from such membranes, the instantaneous "trampoline-like" re-adjustment of the pupil will help to assure the surgeon that all of these vitreous wick bands have been lysed during the laser application. Follow-up with fluorescein angiography (to assess the extent of cystoid macular edema) will also document the success of this procedure where the recuperating vision lags behind the surgical success by some weeks.

YAG lasers may be used to perform anterior capsulotomy hours or days before actual cataract surgery. This allows for lens hydration and facilitates extracapsular cataract extraction. Increased intra-ocular pressure, immune response, or intra-ocular inflammation may result if too much time elapses before cataract extraction is performed. One also wonders if this might not initiate phakolytic glaucoma, which paradoxically seems surprisingly low in our era of extracapsular extraction. One must presume that cortical remnants are always present in the extraordinarily large number of patients who have undergone this procedure. The preliminary procedure is not recommended for patients with glaucoma or for those with hypermature cataract. Advantages to this procedure include the ability to shape the anterior capsulotomy and the possibility of presoftening the nucleus. Photophakal fragmentation refers to the softening of the nucleus with YAG laser bursts before surgical anterior capsulotomy to "avoid" increased intra-ocular pressure and inflammation.

Complications of Laser Surgery

Complications of laser procedures related to surgery are infrequent and usually transitory. Of almost 18,000 cases reported in an FDA study,[7] final visual acuity showed no change or improvement in 96% of cases with a decrease in only 4% of cases. While the rate of complications is extraordinarily low, however, the complications may be clinically significant.

Operative complications include damage to an intra-ocular lens, and even its fracture, as well as rupture of the anterior hyaloid face. The likelihood of pitting and fracturing an intra-ocular lens increases if it is in the posterior chamber position close to the posterior capsule, and if the posterior capsule membrane is thick and fibrous and requires high energy output and a high number of laser bursts. Rupture of the anterior hyaloid face is more common in cases of aphakia than pseudophakia. Other operative complications include corneal edema, which is apparently due to manipulation during the procedure itself, with or without contact lenses, and this has been shown to occur in 0.3% of cases. Various supplementary studies show no change in the endothelial cell count, however.[12] Application of the YAG laser to within 1 mm of the endothelium is very likely to cause damage to endothelial cells and to cause endothelial cell loss, while careful focusing and power selection minimize this risk. This is most likely to occur at synechiolysis or at the application of YAG laser to lyse vitreous wick membranes going through the pupil, often deforming it, and inserting in the original cataract wound.

Since YAG lasers do not cause coagulation of tissue, bleeding can occur if vascularized tissue is inadvertently lysed or when adhesions between an iris and intra-ocular lens are broken, especially when synechiolysis is being achieved. It is not uncommon for bleeding to continue for seemingly endless seconds. Hyphema may result and cause secondary intra-ocular pressure rise. Bleeding may also occur due to shock wave disruption of adjacent iris blood vessels in areas of iridocapsular adhesions. Bleeding, however, usually appears not to be a serious problem and is self-limited in the vast majority of cases. If uncontrolled eye-threatening bleeding occurs, it is advisable to move the patient from the YAG laser to the argon laser and immediately apply argon laser coagulation to the area, thus preventing further problems.

The most frequent and major postoperative complication with YAG laser surgery is an increase in intra-ocular pressure. Aron-Rosa[6] reported an increased pressure in 27% of patients treated with mode locked laser and 46% of those treated with Q-switched YAG laser. Neither group of patients received prophylactic medication beforehand. With such pretreatment therapy, however, the corresponding figures dropped remarkably to 2% and 7% respectively. Brown and co-workers[17] noted that in the majority of eyes, with pressures greater than 30 mm Hg after laser treatment, the pressure peaked between 1 and 3 hours following the procedure. Thus, it is advised to monitor the patient's eye pressure 1 to 2 hours after treatment and before discharge, or to have the patient return the very next day for a repeat pressure check in all cases of YAG laser treatment. In this clinical study, the pressure dropped to less than 22 mm Hg within 24 hours in more than 60% of patients who had YAG laser treatment, and at the end of one week 90% of patients, without treatment, showed no pressure elevation. It has been noted that the elevation of pressure will persist in approximately 2% of patients undergoing YAG laser treatment who, therefore, need to be treated for secondary glaucoma as an ongoing problem. Patients who are predisposed to intra-ocular pressure rise are usually those receiving high total amounts of energy or an extreme amount of laser pulses, or those with pre-existing glaucoma or an inherited tendency to it. These patients might benefit from pretreatment with antiglaucoma medications and careful monitoring of their intra-ocular pressure immediately following laser treatment, especially within the first few hours thereafter. A significantly higher rate of increased intra-ocular pressure follows laser treatment in aphakic patients as opposed to those in psdeudophakic patients.

The incidence of retinal detachment after YAG laser treatment has been reported to be less than 1.25%.[6] Indirect ophthalmoscopy with scleral depression is suggested after YAG laser capsulotomy as well as vitreous band lysis since a relationship may exist between the laser energy and the development of peripheral retinal breaks and their subsequent detachments.

Photocoagulation treatment has long been recognized as effective in reducing the duration of sensory retinal detachment in central serous choroidopathy. A variety of wavelengths have been reported as clinically useful, however, since krypton red is minimally absorbed by the retinal capillary beds, the nerve fiber layer, and the macular xanthophyll pigment, photocoagulation with this wavelength has theoretical and practical advantages for use in the macular area.[39]

References

1. Steinert RF, Puliafito CA: The Neodymmium:YAG Laser in Ophthalmology, Chapter 1. Philadelphia, WB Saunders, 1985
2. Aron-Rosa D: Editorial: Int J Cataract Surg 1:4, 1984
3. Fankenhauser FW, Roussel P, Steffan J: Clinical studies on the efficiency of high power laser radiation upon some structures of the anterior segment. Int Ophthalmol 3:129–139, 1981
4. Mainster M, Ho PC, Mainster CJ: Laser photodisruptors. Ophthalmol 90:360–363, 1983
5. Kelman CD: Neodymmium:YAG laser. Symposium on Cataract Surgery, No 6. New Orleans, Louisiana, 1984

INDEX

The letter f after a page number indicates a figure; t following a page number indicates tabular material.